W9-CBS-960

51 Puppy Tricks

QUARRY

"It's my turn now,
play with me,
I can do it!"

51 Puppy Tricks

Step-by-Step Activities to Engage, Challenge, and Bond with Your Puppy

Kyra Sundance & Jadie

Photography by Nick Saglimbeni

BEVERLY MASSACHUSETTS

QUARRY BOOKS

First published in the United States of America by
Quarry Books, a member of
Quayside Publishing Group
100 Cummings Center
Suite 406-L
Beverly, Massachusetts 01915-6101
Telephone: (978) 282-9590
Fax: (978) 283-2742
www.quarrybooks.com

Library of Congress Cataloging-in-Publication Data is available

ISBN-13: 978-1-59253-571-2
ISBN-10: 1-59253-571-2

10 9 8 7 6 5 4

Design: Sundance MediaCom (www.sundancemediacom.com)
Photography: Nick Saglimbeni (www.slickforce.com)
"Do More With Your Dog!" is a registered trademark of
Kyra Sundance

Printed in China

www.101dogtricks.com

He is your friend, your
partner, your defender,
your dog. You are his life,
his love, his leader. He will
be yours, faithful and true,
to the last beat of his heart.
You owe it to him to be
worthy of such devotion.

—Anonymous

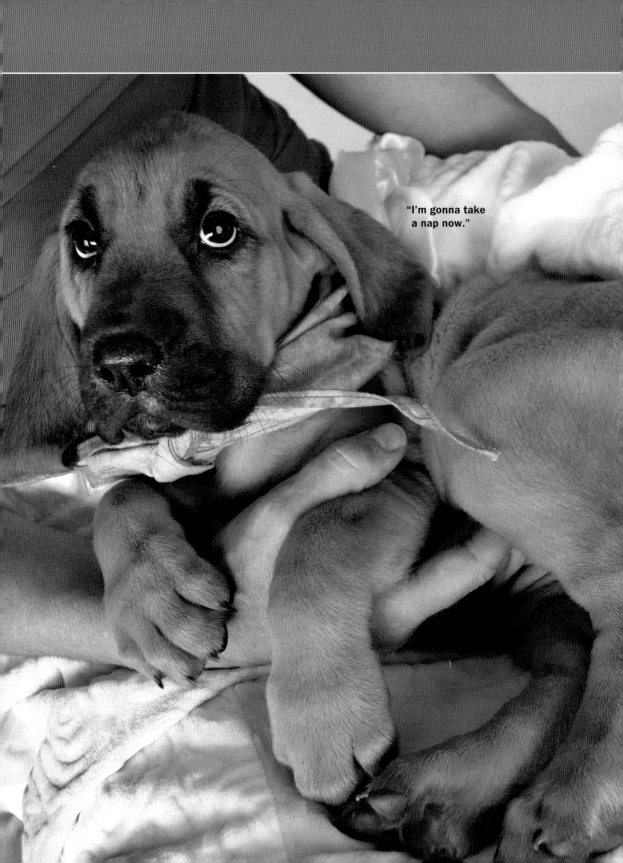

"I'm gonna take a nap now."

CONTENTS

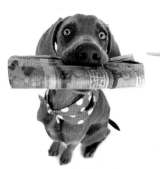
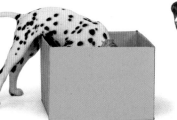
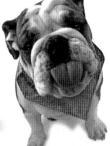
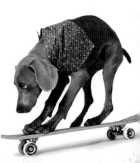

We hope this book inspires you
to not only teach tricks, but to
"Do More With Your Dog!®"

— Kyra Sundance & Jadie

*Do More
With Your Dog!*®
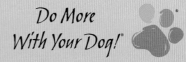

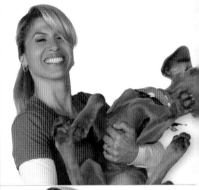

When you bring a new puppy into your household, he becomes part of your family. By making the effort to work with your puppy on his first tricks, you're taking a strong step toward developing a closer bond with your dog.

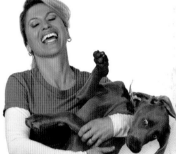

In this book you will use positive training methods to build a joyful relationship with your puppy, where he is a willing partner in the training process. Trick training builds relationships by deepening communication pathways, trust, and mutual respect. It offers a way to bond with your puppy as you strive toward common goals and delight in your successes. The trust and cooperative spirit developed through this process will last a lifetime.

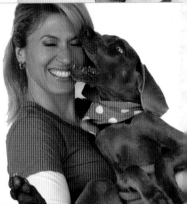

Measure your puppy's success not only by the tricks he has learned, but also by improved attention and focus. Not all puppies will learn at the same rate, but remember, he's *your* puppy and his success need only be measured in *your* eyes. While it's motivating to have a goal of a finished trick, the best thing that comes out of training your puppy is the bond that develops through working together. Don't be so focused on the goal that you miss the joys of the journey!

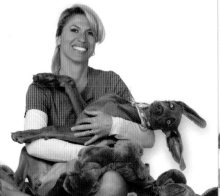

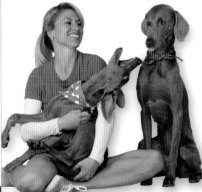

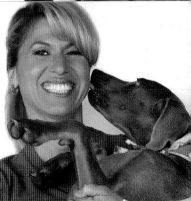

"I have so much
to do today, I
don't know how I
can possibly get
it all done!"

INTRODUCTION

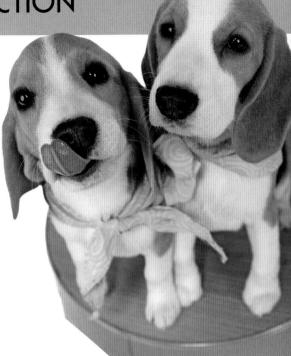

MAKE TRAINING FUN FOR YOUR PUPPY

Teaching tricks to your puppy will increase his intelligence as his brain is challenged to learn new things. Early training will set the tone for how your puppy feels about training in the future, so it is important to keep training fun and rewarding for your puppy.

Don't treat training like a chore or your puppy will associate training, and you, with boredom. Be happy, enthusiastic, and encouraging! Blur the line between play and work by playing a few minutes after every training session.

When your puppy does something right, use your high-pitched "happy voice," which is instinctively rewarding for him. Your happy voice should rise in pitch at the end, in a sing-songy tone: "good boy!"

Don't Show Frustration

Your puppy needs time to learn, and requires many, many consistent repetitions. When teaching him a new trick, your puppy may squirm, paw, and obsess over the treat in your hand. If you feel yourself getting angry or frustrated during a training session, the best thing you can do is to walk away. Your puppy can sense when you are upset, and you wouldn't want him to associate training with your frustration.

Keep Sessions Short

Puppies have short attention spans. Don't train past the point where your puppy has lost interest. Several five-minute sessions per day are ideal for most puppies.

Quit With Him Wanting More

Quit your training session while everyone is having a good time, and before your puppy gets bored or tired. Quit with him wanting more so he looks forward to the next session.

End on a High Note

Keep your puppy feeling good about training by always ending on a successful note, even if you have to go back to an easier step to achieve this. Ask your puppy for a behavior he knows well; praise him excitedly for it; and end the session then.

PUPPY BASICS

HOW OLD IS A "PUPPY" IN THIS BOOK?

The tricks in this book are intended for puppies eight weeks to two years old. There are no prerequisites for trick training. Young puppies should start with the "easy" tricks.

HOW LONG DOES IT TAKE TO TRAIN A PUPPY?

The more tricks your puppy learns, the quicker he'll pick up new ones. Each trick in this book has a section on "what to expect" during the learning process. It generally takes a hundred repetitions for a puppy to learn a trick. Different puppies will learn in different ways, and at different speeds, so don't be frustrated if you aren't seeing the results you want right away.

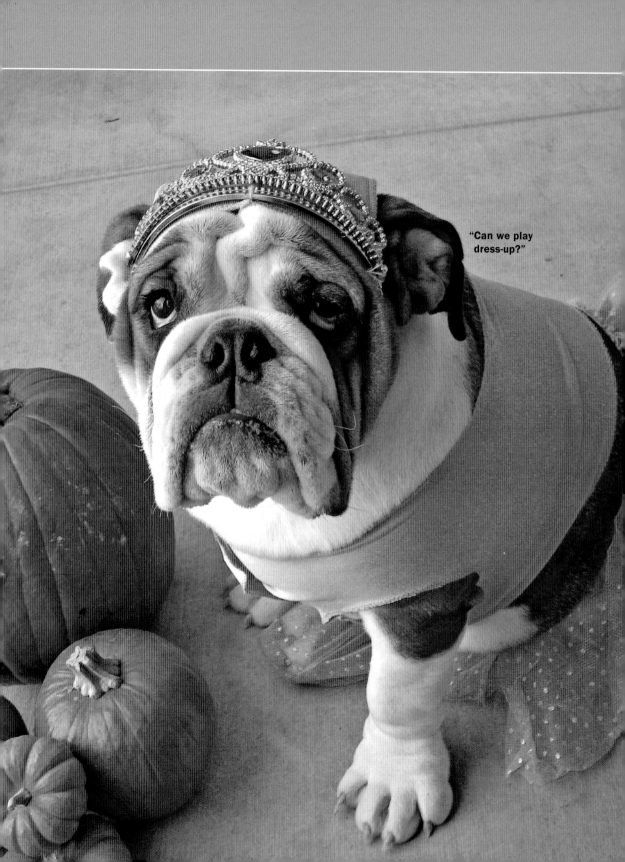

"Can we play dress-up?"

PUPPIES LEARN THROUGH POSITIVE REINFORCEMENT

Positive reinforcement training methods are the easiest and most effective way to teach a trick to your puppy. Positive reinforcement is the rewarding of good behavior; you get your puppy to do a trick, you give him a reward, and he learns to repeat the trick.

Positive reinforcement methods strengthen the relationship between you and your puppy as you work collaboratively in an encouraging, stress-free and fear-free environment. Your puppy participates in the learning process with a positive attitude, and enjoys working with you. The trust and cooperative spirit developed through positive reinforcement training will last a lifetime.

Treats as Rewards

Although a reward for a puppy can be a toy, play, or praise, we usually use food treat. Treats are a high-value reward that can be dispensed quickly. Keep your puppy extra motivated by using "people food" treats, such as chicken, steak, cheese, goldfish crackers, noodles, or meatballs. Use pea-sized, soft, tasty treats that your puppy can swallow easily.

Try microwaving hot dog slices on a paper-towel-covered plate for three minutes for a tasty treat!

Reward Success, Ignore the Rest

One of the key skills your puppy develops through trick training is his ability to problem-solve through experimentation. Encourage your puppy to try a lot of behaviors, and let him know (with a treat) which ones were correct.

When a puppy offers a behavior that is not correct, it is best to ignore his unsuccessful attempt rather than punishing it. If you were to say "no" every time your puppy offered an incorrect behavior, your puppy would become reluctant to try anything at all. Most puppies would rather do nothing than to be wrong.

Instill an enthusiasm for training in your puppy by building his esteem and his motivation. By focusing on the positive, you will help your puppy to be successful.

Calming an Overly Excited Puppy

Sometimes a puppy becomes so excited during training that you need to get him to calm down and regain focus. Do this by silently putting your arms at your sides and looking away for a few seconds. This will inform your puppy (without reprimanding or frustrating him) that he is not on a path that will lead to a reward, and he needs to give you his calm attention. A few seconds is usually enough for him calm down a bit, at which time you can resume your training. Repeat this process every time your puppy gets too hyper.

"I'm a good girl . . . most of the time."

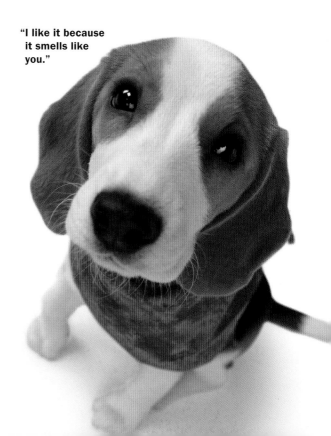

Click

PUPPY TRAINING TECHNIQUES

We use different techniques to train a puppy than we use to train a dog. Puppies are softer than adult dogs, and they are not as familiar with human speech and actions. If you have trained adult dogs before, you'll want to adjust your technique for your puppy.

Lure, Don't Manipulate

There are two obvious ways to get a puppy into a desired position: You can lure him by encouraging him to follow a treat, or you can assert physical pressure to manipulate him into position. It is tempting to manipulate your puppy's body physically because it is faster and more precise; however, it can actually delay the learning process. By manipulating your puppy, you are encouraging him to relinquish initiative and be led. He is not required to engage his brain and is not learning the motor skills necessary to position his body himself. When possible, it is always preferable to lure your puppy to position his body himself.

Timing

During the learning process, your puppy may squirm and try a variety of different things. You need to let him immediately know if each thing he tried was a success (treat) or nonsuccess (no treat). The key to helping him understand the goal behavior is to give him the treat at the exact moment that he performed correctly. Be ready with a treat in your hand, and release it the instant your puppy performs correctly. Don't reward five seconds after he has done the behavior, as your puppy may not understand what he did to earn the reward. The key to teaching any trick is to reward success at the instant the puppy performs correctly.

Marker Training and Clickers

It can sometimes be logistically difficult to reward your puppy at the exact moment he performed correctly. If your puppy is learning to jump through a hoop, for example, you wouldn't be able to give him a treat at the exact moment he intersects the hoop.

But you *can* use a specific word or sound at that exact moment to let your puppy know the instant he earned his reward. We call this special sound a **reward marker**. A reward marker is always quickly followed by a treat.

In dog training, a **clicker** is commonly used to make the reward marker sound. A clicker is a handheld gadget with a metal tongue that makes a *click-click* sound when pressed.

You can use a unique word (such as "good!" or "click!") to be your reward marker sound, however a clicker tends to work better than a word for puppy training. Puppies haven't yet had the experience of differentiating your words, and therefore your unique word won't be as distinct for him as the clicker sound. The clicker also has the advantages of being short, crisp, and consistent—it sounds exactly the same every time. (Train your puppy to **respond to a clicker** with the trick on page 20.)

"I like it because it smells like you."

PROGRESSION AND REGRESSION

A puppy learns when he gets it right, and gets a treat. A puppy doesn't learn anything from unsuccessful attempts. So as a trainer, you need to help him get as many successful attempts as possible. Do this by setting the criteria for success very low. Reward small baby steps in the learning process so that your puppy has lots and lots of success.

Upping the Ante

When your puppy is first learning, give him a treat for just the smallest baby step toward a goal behavior. As your puppy progresses, you will start asking more of him to earn the treat. In this way we gradually refine a rudimentary behavior into a more extreme version. We call this **upping the ante**.

When first teaching a puppy to shake a paw, you reward him for barely lifting his paw. Once he has the hang of this, you up the ante and withhold the treat until he lifts his paw higher, or holds it longer.

The rule of thumb: every time your puppy achieves a step with about 75 percent success, it is time to up the ante and demand a higher skill to earn the treat.

Regression is Part of Progression

The key to keeping your puppy motivated is to keep him challenged, and achieving regular successes. Try not to let your puppy be wrong more than two or three times in a row, or he could become discouraged and not wish to perform. If your puppy is struggling, temporarily lower the criteria for success. Regress back to an easier step where he can be successful for a while.

The process of learning a behavior is not linear. Your puppy will go through numerous spurts of learning and regression. Don't be reluctant to go back a step—it's usually only needed for a short while, and will give your puppy confidence to move forward. Never push ahead in the training process if you reach a point where your puppy is not confident. Instead, back up a few steps to where your puppy showed the greatest degree of confidence and build his skills from there.

HOW TO USE THIS BOOK

Start anywhere! Each trick displays a difficulty rating, tips, troubleshooting answers, and a "what to expect" section that gives an estimate on how long the trick will take to teach. You can work on several new tricks within the same training session.

Should I Use the Verbal Cue or the Hand Signal?

Where applicable, both the verbal cue and corresponding hand signal for a trick are indicated in this book. Over time your puppy will learn to respond to either one. Most puppies actually respond more readily to the hand signal than to the verbal cue.

The cues and hand signals shown in this book are industry standards. Although the hand signals may look arbitrary, they have often evolved from the luring gestures used in the puppy's initial training. The raising of your hand as a signal to "sit" evolves from your initial upward baiting gesture. A downward hand motion is used to signal "down," and parallels your initial baiting of your puppy near the floor. And the flick of your wrist to the right is a diminished version of the large circle you drew when teaching your puppy to "spin."

Let's Start Training!

You're on your way to a wonderful, exciting adventure with your new puppy. Grab your treat bag, your puppy's favorite toy, your copy of 51 Puppy Tricks . . . and let's get started!

"My owner says
I'm special
because I have
freckles."

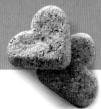

TRAINING GEAR

A few items of proper training gear will make your sessions go more smoothly.

Food Treats

Use soft, tasty, pea-sized food treats that your puppy can swallow quickly.

Treat Bag

Pet stores sell treat bags (also called bait bags) that clip onto your pants. These give you quick access to treats without having to dig in your pockets.

Short Tab Lead

A tab lead is a short line with no loop at the end (so that your puppy's paw won't get caught in it.) It hangs from your puppy's collar, but is short enough so that it does not get in the way of his movement. A tab lead allows you to train your puppy off-leash, while still having a way to hold him when you need to.

Clicker

In this book you will use a clicker as a reward marker to teach some of the tricks. The clicker sound lets your puppy know when he is correct. Inexpensive clickers can be purchased at most pet stores.

A Good Attitude!

The most important training tool of all is your praise and encouragement!

**TOP 10
PUPPY TRAINING TIPS:**

1. Use tasty treats.
2. Give a treat the instant your puppy performs the correct behavior.
3. If you can't give a treat at that instant, click your clicker and follow up with a treat.
4. Motivate—use your happy voice.
5. Train in short five-minute sessions.
6. Reward success and ignore the rest.
7. Be consistent.
8. End the session with your puppy wanting more.
9. Be patient—it won't happen overnight.
10. Be a fun person to be around!

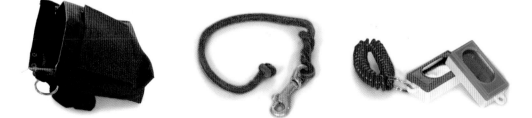

Chapter 1:

Preliminary Skills

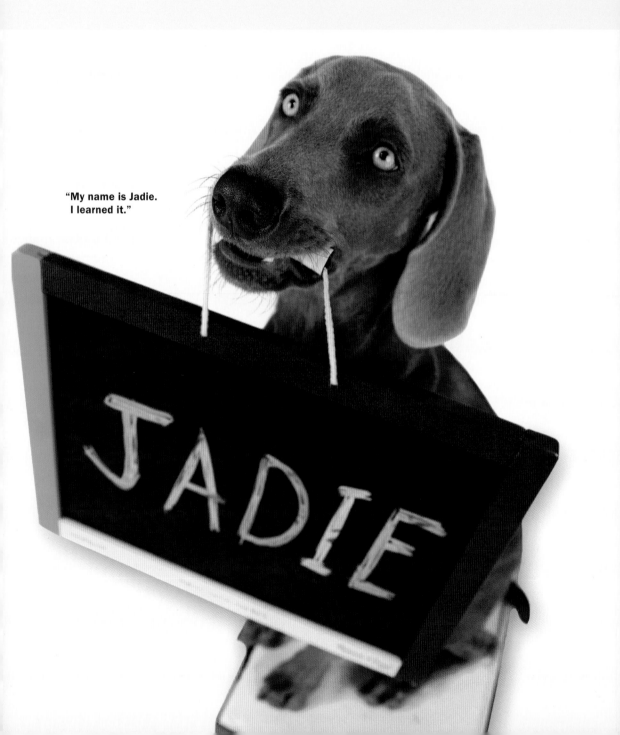

"My name is Jadie.
I learned it."

Start your puppy off right by teaching her the training

fundamentals. The tricks in this chapter teach your puppy to focus on you and to perform basic behaviors. These tricks introduce your puppy to the concept of positive reinforcement, and of responding to your cues in order to earn rewards. These preliminary skills will establish a pattern for your puppy's ability to learn for the rest of her life.

In this chapter, your puppy will learn to respond to a clicker, to give you attention by looking into your eyes, and to control her movements.

There will be times while you are teaching these preliminary skills that you will need to get your puppy's attention. Teach your puppy her name, so that you can ask for her attention. Teach her by saying her name in a happy, high-pitched tone, which will encourage her to look at you. When she does, give her a treat, praise, or do something fun such as toss a toy!

Hearing her name should elicit a positive feeling for your puppy. She should respond to it with enthusiasm, never hesitancy or fear. Use your puppy's name in conjunction with praise, and at times when she is calm, confident, and attentive.

Don't use your puppy's name in conjunction with reprimands or when she is in a stressful situation, scared, or aggressive.

Respond to a Clicker

A clicker device can become a valuable tool in puppy training. In order to take advantage of this tool, you must first teach your puppy to respond to its sound. Do so by building the association between the clicker sound and the food reward. This is called "charging up the clicker."

"I like treats!"

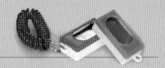

1 A clicker is a handheld thumb-sized box with a metal tongue that makes a click-click sound when pressed. Clickers are widely available at pet stores. Use a flexible strap or rubber band to attach it to your wrist for easy access.

2 Put about twenty small treats in your pocket or your treat bag. Walk around casually near your puppy, but do not give any instruction to her. Occasionally, and at random intervals, click your clicker.

3 After clicking, immediately give a treat to your puppy. Try to give the treat within two seconds of clicking, to help your puppy develop the association between the two events.

WHAT TO EXPECT: It doesn't take long before that click sound makes your puppy's head spin toward you—which indicates she has formed the association. Within a few minutes (and maybe twenty clicks), your puppy should be responding to the clicker, and will be ready to start training tricks with this tool.

TROUBLESHOOTING

I'M NOT SURE WHEN TO CLICK

At this stage, the goal is merely to build the association between the *click-click* sound and the food treat. There is no wrong time to click. The important thing is to give the treat immediately after each click.

TIP! Once puppy has learned to respond to a clicker, you can use this tool in training. There are three rules to using a clicker:

1. Click to mark any behavior you wish encourage.
2. Click the *instant* the correct behavior happens.
3. Each click is followed by a treat (no multiple clicks).

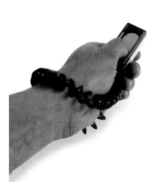

1 Attach a wrist strap to your clicker for easy access.

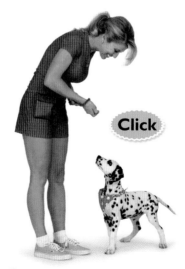

2 Randomly click your clicker.

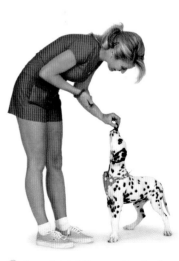

3 Immediately follow up with a treat.

Touch My Hand

Teach your puppy to touch your hand with his nose. This skill will come in handy in getting your puppy to come to you.

"I get brushed every day and sometimes I get a bath if I roll in stuff."

TEACH IT:

1 Hold your clicker in one hand. In your other hand, hold a treat between your fingers, and hold your hand flat, with your palm toward your puppy. Get your puppy's attention as you do this by saying "cookie" or whichever word he understands to mean a treat.

2 Encourage your puppy to investigate the treat by saying "touch!" in an encouraging voice.

3 The instant you feel his nose touch your hand, click your clicker to let him know that was the behavior that earned him the treat. Allow him to take the treat from your hand. Repeat this exercise a few times.

4 Now try it without a treat held between your fingers. Hold out your hand and say "touch!" The instant your puppy touches your hand, click your clicker, and then give him a treat from your pocket.

WHAT TO EXPECT: Practice ten iterations per day and within a few days your puppy will learn this trick!

TROUBLESHOOTING

MY PUPPY IS MORE INTERESTED IN MY POCKET WITH THE TREATS THAN IN TOUCHING MY HAND
Go back to holding a treat between your fingers to regain his focus on your hand. If this doesn't work, try storing your treats in a bowl on a nearby counter, where they are out of his reach, but still easily accessible by you.

TIP! Did your puppy run off? Hold out your hand and call "touch!" to see him race back to you!

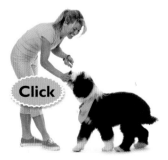

1 Show your puppy a treat held between your fingers.

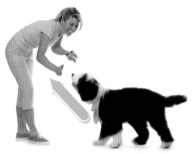

2 Encourage your puppy by saying "touch!"

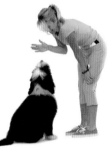

Click

3 Click the instant your puppy's nose touches your hand, and allow him to take the treat.

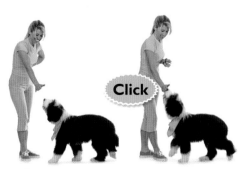

Click

4 Now try it without a treat held between your fingers. Click when he touches your hand.

Watch Me

When you have your puppy's eyes, you have his attention. Teach your puppy to look directly into your eyes as a way to ask for his attention.

"Play with me, play with me, play with me . . ."

TEACH IT:

1. Kneel down to puppy height. Hold your clicker in one hand, and in the other hold a treat at your puppy's eye level.

2. Slowly bring the treat back toward your eyes, while using a calm, drawn-out voice to cue "focus . . . focus . . . "

3. Once your puppy holds eye contact for a second or two, click your clicker, and give him the treat. You want your puppy to be successful, so try to click before he loses interest and looks away. As he gets better, you can start to require longer stares before you click.

4. Begin to phase out the handheld treat and instead use your pointed finger between your eyes and the word "focus" to cue his stare. Click when he makes eye contact and give him a treat.

WHAT TO EXPECT: A puppy's eyesight is not fully developed until he is about nine months old, so very young puppies will be less able to focus on your eyes. Shy puppies may be hesitant to look into your eyes, possibly because they feel it is confrontational. This exercise will be especially helpful for those timid puppies. Most puppies can learn to make eye contact within a couple of days.

TROUBLESHOOTING

MY PUPPY WON'T LOOK INTO MY EYES
Sit on the ground, at puppy height, to appear less domineering. Speak gently, and practice daily. Let your puppy make the decision on his own to look into your eyes—do not force the exercise.

TIP! Make a habit of requiring a moment of calm attention before routine rewards, such as at the front door before taking your puppy on a walk, or at the food dish before chowtime. As soon as your puppy holds eye contact for a second or two, click and give him his reward. This will teach your puppy self-control, and that calm, attentive behavior is rewarded.

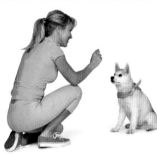

1. Get your puppy's attention with a treat.

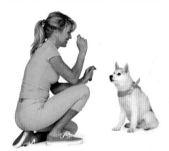

2. Slowly move the treat toward your eyes, as you say "focus."

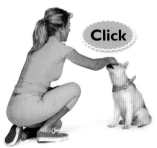

3. Once your puppy holds eye contact, click, and give him the treat.

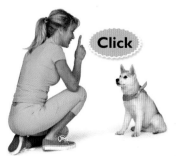

4. Use your pointed finger to cue this behavior.

Settle

"I did good today."

Teach your puppy to settle calmly. This will accustom her to being restrained, and is useful in grooming and examining your puppy.

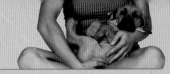

TEACH IT:

1 Choose a time when your puppy is tired and calm. Pick her up gently and cradle her on her back in your arms. Hold her securely and sit on the floor or a bed as you do this, so that your puppy won't fall if she accidently squirms from your arms. Stroke her gently to make this experience a pleasurable one. Say "settle" in a soft, pleasant voice.

2 Another way to do the settle exercise is to lay your puppy on her back on your extended legs. Pick her up facing you, and slowly roll her back onto your legs. If your puppy squirms, gently keep her on her back until she relaxes. Do not increase pressure, but stay calm and consistent. If you wait long enough, she will eventually relax. Once she relaxes, relax your hold on her.

WHAT TO EXPECT: Puppies vary widely on how they tolerate being restrained. In the beginning, just have your puppy settle for a few seconds, and then praise her and release her. As she becomes more accustomed to this exercise, try to have her settle for twenty seconds.

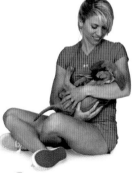

1 Cradle your puppy on her back.

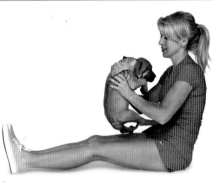

2 Pick your puppy up facing you.

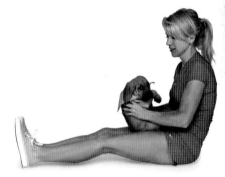

Set your puppy on your legs.

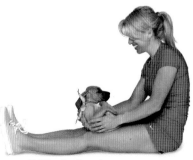

Roll her backward.

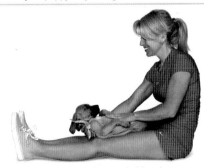

Once she relaxes, relax your hold on her.

When told to "kennel up," your puppy goes happily into his crate.

"Sometimes I like to sleep in my kennel and sometimes I don't wanna sleep and then I bark."

TEACH IT:

1 A crate provides a den for your puppy, which instinctually feels safe to him. Your puppy's kennel is his personal space and he deserves to be left alone while inside. Blankets and a cover make it cozy and comfortable, and a few toys inside will make it fun.

2 Allow your puppy to approach and explore a new kennel on his own. Once he is comfortable with his crate, toss a treat inside as you tell him to "kennel up." Praise him for going inside.

3 Now that he looks forward to this command, tell him to "kennel up" without tossing a treat inside. Once he goes in the crate, immediately praise him and give him a treat. Remember to give the treat while he is inside the kennel, as this is the position you wish to reinforce.

4 You can give your puppy a Kong toy filled with peanut butter to keep him busy and happy in his kennel.

WHAT TO EXPECT: As part of his bedtime routine, your puppy will look forward to kenneling up and receiving his good-night treat.

TROUBLESHOOTING

MY PUPPY WON'T GO IN HIS CRATE
You don't want to ever force your puppy into his crate, or he may resist it thereafter. Be patient and allow him time to explore it on his own. Puppies will show significantly less fear of an object if allowed to approach it on their own, as opposed to being forced toward it.

TIP! Your puppy's crate should be large enough for him to stand up, turn around and lie down comfortably.

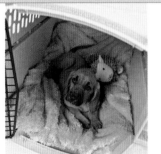

1 Blankets and a toy will make his kennel cozy.

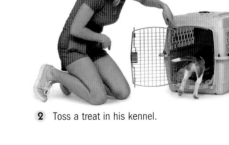

2 Toss a treat in his kennel.

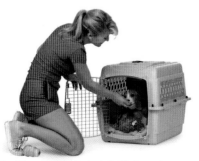

3 Give him a treat while he is in his kennel.

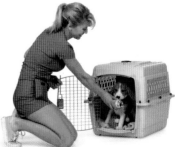

4 A food toy will keep him busy and happy in his kennel.

Come

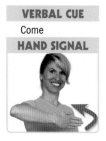

"I have a friend
and he's a cat
and sometimes
he scratches."

Upon your call, your puppy
comes immediately to you.
Always reward your puppy
for obeying your "come"
command, whether it be
with praise, a treat, or a
play session.

TEACH IT:

1 Most puppies will eagerly come to you when called, so puppyhood is the perfect time to teach this trick. Say "come," and entice your puppy to come to you by crouching down, acting excited, patting your legs, and opening your arms.

2 When your puppy comes to you, have a party! Give him a treat and tell him how wonderful he is!

3 Engage your puppy's chase drive by calling "come" and running away from him. Reward him excitedly when he catches you. Remember, catching you is your puppy's reward, so make it fun for him when he does!

4 Now it's time to transition your training from a game to a command. Put your puppy on a lead and tell him to "come." If he does not come to you on his own, use the lead to reel him in to you. In both cases, give him a treat when he gets to you.

WHAT TO EXPECT: A puppy can learn the meaning of "come" within a week. Keep this command happy, and reward your puppy every single time he comes (even if the reward is just praise or a petting).

TROUBLESHOOTING

MY PUPPY RUNS OFF!
Do not chase your puppy, as that will only encourage him to play keep-away. Act interested in something on the ground, or toss a toy around and act interested in it. That should pique your puppy's curiosity and get him to return to you.

TIP! Only call your puppy to "come" for good things, and never for bad things (such as a bath or nail trimming). This will keep him eager to come to you!

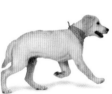
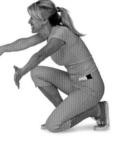

1 Pat your legs, open your arms, and call "come."

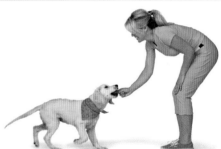

2 Reward your puppy profusely when he reaches you.

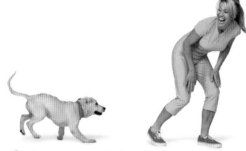

3 Engage your puppy's chase drive by running away from him.

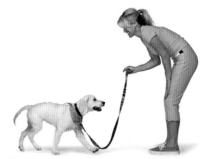

4 Transition from a game to a command, by enforcing the behavior with a lead.

Stay

VERBAL CUE

Stay

HAND SIGNAL

"You're funny when you do that!"

When in a stay, your puppy holds her current position until released. A puppy can learn a sit-stay, a down-stay, or even a stand-stay.

TEACH IT:

1. Start with your puppy sitting. Stand directly in front of her, holding your palm in front of her nose. In a firm tone, say "stay."

2. Take a step backward, while keeping your hand up. Look directly into your puppy's eyes to hold her in place. Wait one second, then step forward. Praise your puppy with "good stay" and give her a treat. Be sure to give the praise and treat while your puppy is sitting, and not after she has stood up.

3. If your puppy moves from her stay before you have released her, put her back in the spot where she was told to stay.

4. Gradually increase the time you ask your puppy to stay, as well as the distance between yourselves. You want your puppy to be successful so if she is breaking her stays, regress to a time and distance she is able to achieve.

WHAT TO EXPECT: Puppies need time to learn self-control. Ask your puppy only for what she is able to achieve. As she matures, she will be better able to hold a longer stay.

TROUBLESHOOTING

MY PUPPY KEEPS GETTING UP
Use very little verbal communication when teaching this skill. Talking evokes action, and you want inaction. Use slow and deliberate movements.

MY PUPPY BREAKS HER STAY A SECOND BEFORE I RELEASE HER
Do not show her the treat until you give it to her, as it may pull her forward. Vary your pattern; sometimes return to her and leave her again without rewarding.

TIP! Use your puppy's name when you want to prompt action ("Molly, come!") Do not use her name when you want inaction ("stay").

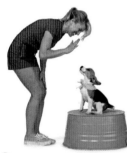

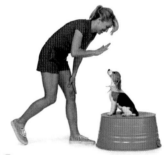

1 Command "stay" and hold up your hand.

2 Take a step backward, keeping your hand up.

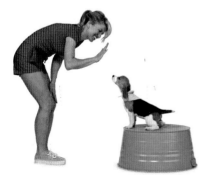

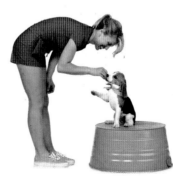

Hold your puppy with your eyes.

Step forward and reward your puppy.

Find Me

Hide from your puppy, call for her to find you by name, and reward her when she does. This game teaches your puppy to recognize your name, and also conditions her to think of *you* as a reward.

"I'm really good at finding stuff, and once I found this great thing in the yard."

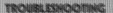

TEACH IT:

1 Make this game fun for your puppy with high energy and laughter! Put some treats in your pocket and when your puppy is distracted, slip out of the room.

2 In a happy voice call "find [your name]!" Listen for your puppy's footsteps, and if you do not hear her running toward you, call again.

3 When your puppy finds you, throw a party! Laugh, praise her, and give her a treat. Reinforce her recognition of your name by saying "good find [your name]!"

WHAT TO EXPECT: This trick is a wonderful combination of fun and learning! Most puppies love this game and will be super excited to find you! As your puppy's sense of smell matures, she will use her nose to sniff you out, and you'll need to find more difficult hiding spots!

TROUBLESHOOTING

MY PUPPY GETS ANXIOUS AND WHINES WHEN SHE CAN'T FIND ME

If your puppy is looking for you, but can't find you, she may become anxious. Help her out by clapping or moving a little so she can detect you. Her victory will be that much sweeter if it was a little challenging to find you!

TIP! Help your puppy learn the names of other family members as well, by having them hide and instructing your puppy to find them by name.

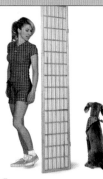

1 Sneak out of the room when your puppy is distracted.

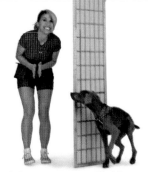

2 Call to your puppy to "find [your name]!"

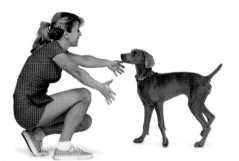

3 Throw a party when your puppy finds you!

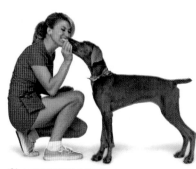

Give your puppy a treat.

Chapter 2:

Body Positions

"Oops! Wait, let me do it again, are you watching?"

Paws, legs, heads, and mouths can be structured into a variety of body positions, and your puppy can learn a name for each position. Teach your puppy a name for raising his paw, sitting, or rolling over. Learning names for these positions will give you and your puppy a common language in which to communicate.

Some of the tricks in this chapter require physical strength and coordination that a young puppy may not yet have. Crawling, bowing, and rolling over will be more difficult for a puppy than learning a sit, a down, or lifting his paw. Some tricks, such as barking or singing, will come easier for a confident and well-socialized puppy.

Although it may be tempting to physically manipulate your puppy's body into position, such as by lifting his paw while teaching him to shake hands, it will benefit him more if you allow him the time to figure out the body position on his own.

We often use the technique of luring the puppy's head in order to get him to position himself. This technique is very effective when executed properly. Study the photos in order to help you position and move the treat at the proper angle.

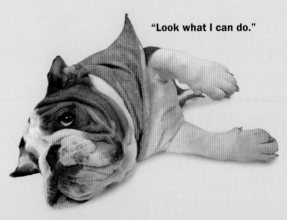

"Look what I can do."

Sit

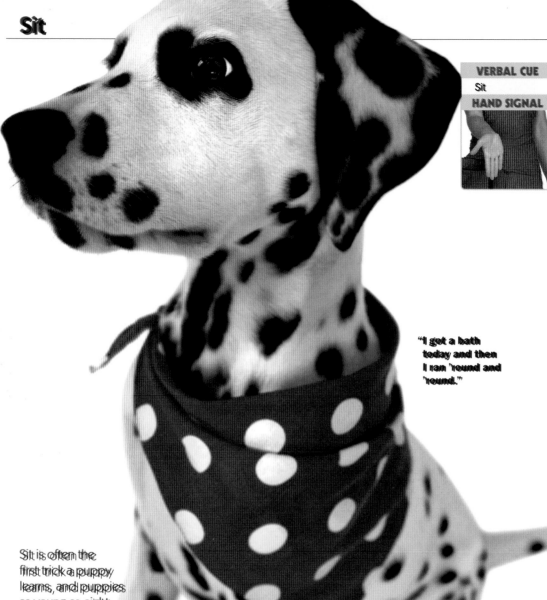

"I got a bath
today and then
I ran 'round and
'round."

Sit is often the
first trick a puppy
learns, and puppies
as young as eight
weeks can learn
this trick.

1. Kneel in front of your puppy. Hold your clicker in one hand, and in the other hold a treat in front of your puppy's nose.

2. Say "sit" and slowly move the treat in an arc, up and back over your puppy's head. This should cause her nose to point up and her rear to drop. There is a little trick to this: first lure her nose to point high up, and then start to move the treat down at an angle, from her nose toward her tail.

3. The instant her rear touches the floor, click your clicker and release the treat.

4. If you find your puppy is jumping, it may be that you are holding your treat too high. If your puppy keeps moving backward, it may be that you are moving the the treat horizontally, instead of in an arc.

5. Once your puppy is consistently sitting, wait a few seconds before clicking and rewarding.

WHAT TO EXPECT: Most puppies start to learn this trick within a few days, although it usually takes about 100 repetitions before they can do it consistently.

TROUBLESHOOTING

I CAN'T GET MY PUPPY TO SIT

Some puppies are squirmy, and it may take a while for your puppy to finally sit. Sometimes working in front of a wall will help, as your puppy won't have room to move backward.

TIP! Remember to only reward your puppy while she is in the correct position—sitting.

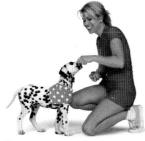

1. Hold a treat in front of your puppy's nose.

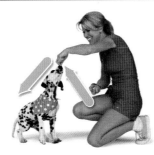

2. Lure her nose up and back, causing her rear to drop.

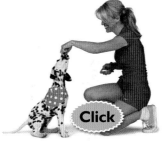

3. Click and reward when her rear touches the floor.

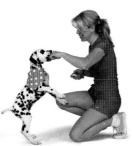

4. Don't hold the treat too high. Don't push the treat horizontally.

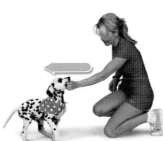

5. Tell your puppy to "sit," and wait a few seconds before clicking and rewarding.

Down

VERBAL CUE
Down

HAND SIGNAL

"I like ice cubes and I like to play with them and I like to crunch them."

Teach your puppy to lie down (if only for a moment). This trick can be learned by very young puppies.

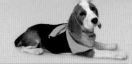

1. Kneel next to your puppy. Show him a treat and move it relatively quickly at down and toward his front paws.

2. When your puppy follows the treat, his nose will end up between his paws, putting him in an awkward position, which will usually make him lie down. If your puppy does not lie down right away, move the treat along the floor toward him, putting him in an even more awkward position. It may take a little time, but your puppy should eventually lie down.

3. The instant your puppy lies down, click your clicker and release the treat.

4. After some practice, try using just your pointed finger on the ground, instead of the treat. When you puppy lies down, click your clicker and give him a treat from your pocket. Remember to give the reward while your puppy is lying down, and not after he has stood up.

WHAT TO EXPECT: Puppies often take two or three weeks to learn this trick. Remember to click your clicker at the exact instant that your puppy lies down, as this will help him understand what he did to earn the treat.

TROUBLESHOOTING

MY PUPPY LIES DOWN ON SOME SURFACES BUT NOT OTHERS
Pay attention to the ground surface. Short-coated puppies will often resist lying down on hard or cold floor. Try a carpet or blanket.

TIP! Practice when your puppy is a little tired, as he will be more inclined to lie down.

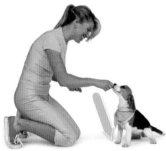

1. Move the treat at an angle toward your puppy's paws.

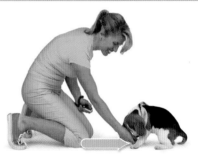

2. Move the treat along the floor toward your puppy.

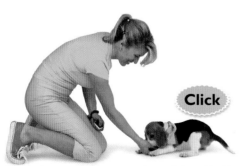

3. The instant your puppy goes down, click, and let him have the treat.

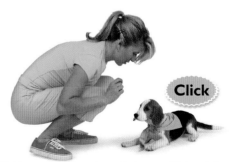

4. Try a pointed finger instead of a treat. Click and give a treat from your pocket.

Crawl

Crawl

"The grass tickles my belly!"

In this trick, your puppy crawls forward, sliding her belly on the floor.

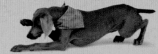

TEACH IT:

1. Start with your puppy lying down, and kneel next to her. Show her a treat hidden under your hand.

2. In a drawn-out voice tell her "crawl . . . " as you slowly slide the treat away from her.

3. She will hopefully take a crawl step or two with her front paws in an effort to follow the treat. Click your clicker when she does this, and let her have the treat.

4. Build up distance by waiting until your puppy takes several crawl steps before clicking and treating.

WHAT TO EXPECT: Many puppies are able to begin crawling in their first training session. Lankier breeds will have a harder time crawling, and all puppies will need to build up strength to crawl farther.

TROUBLESHOOTING

MY PUPPY STANDS UP
You are sliding the treat too fast.

MY PUPPY DOESN'T MOVE
She might be unsure of what she is supposed to do. Keep your energy enthusiastic.

TIP! Your puppy will be more willing to crawl on a comfortable surface such as grass or carpet.

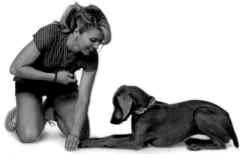

1. Show your puppy a treat hidden under your hand.

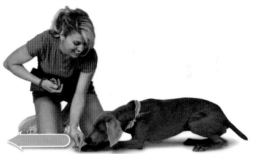

2. Slowly slide the treat away from her.

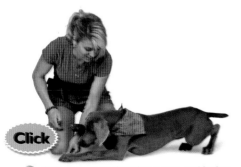

3. Click as soon as she takes a step, and let her have the treat.

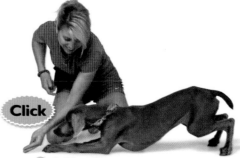

4. Build up distance.

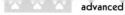
Roll Over

Your puppy rolls sideways on her back, completing a full rotation. Small breed puppies sometimes have an easier time with this behavior, but all puppies are capable of learning this trick.

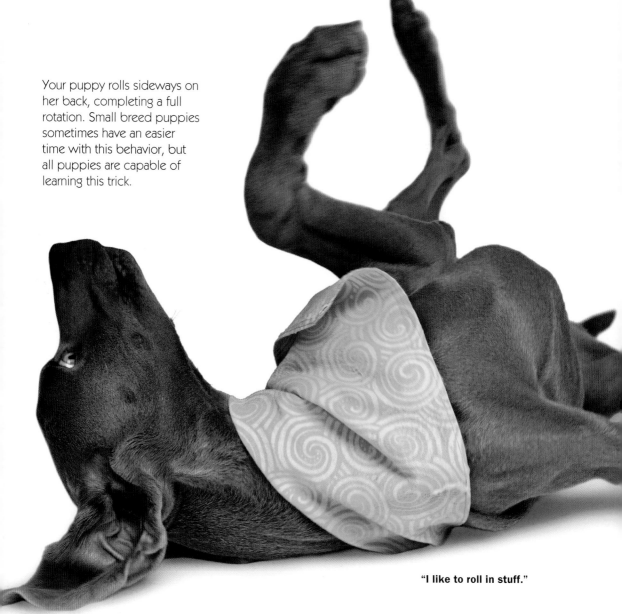

"I like to roll in stuff."

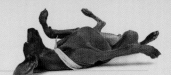

1. Kneel down, facing your puppy as she is lying down. Hold a treat in front of her nose, and move it to the side of her head opposite the direction you wish her to roll.

2. Continue to move the treat toward her shoulder blade. This should lure your puppy to flop onto her side. Click your clicker at that instant and release the treat.

3. When you are ready to move to the next step, continue the motion with your hand as you move the treat from her shoulder blade toward her backbone. This should lure her to roll onto her back, and over to her other side. Click and reward the moment she lands on her opposite side.

4. As she improves, say "roll over" and use a more subtle hand gesture. It often helps to lean your body in the direction of the roll over, to remind your puppy of what she is supposed to do.

WHAT TO EXPECT: Practice five to ten times per session, and in two weeks your puppy could be rolling over!

TROUBLESHOOTING

MY PUPPY IS SQUIRMING, BUT NOT ROLLING ONTO HER SIDE

It's all about your hand position. You want her neck arched as if her nose were trying to touch her shoulder blade.

MY PUPPY ROLLS TO HER SIDE, BUT DOES NOT CONTINUE TO ROLL ONTO HER BACK

Help your puppy finish the roll over by gently guiding her front legs over with your hand.

TIP! This trick will be harder for stocky dogs with short necks, such as bulldogs.

"I go potty outside. Most times."

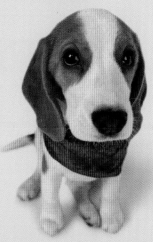

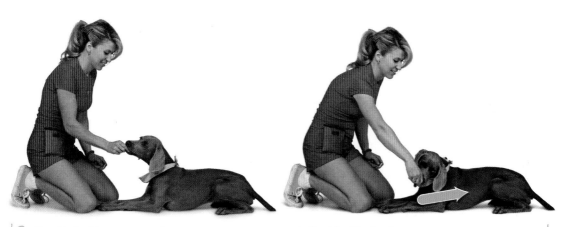

1. Move the treat from your puppy's nose . . .   to the side of her head.

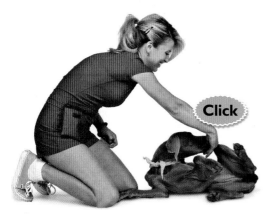

2. Continue to move the treat toward her shoulder blade.

Click

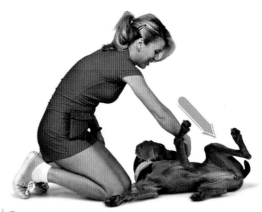

3. Move the treat from her shoulder blade to her backbone.

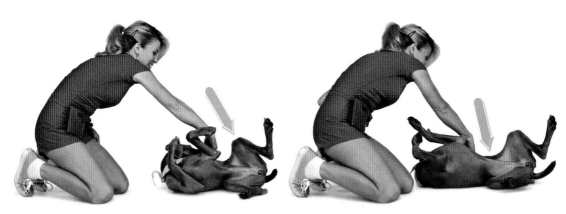

Following the lure, she should roll onto her back . . .

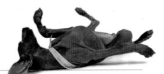

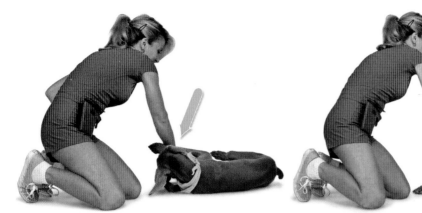

and then onto her other side.

Click and reward when she lands on her side.

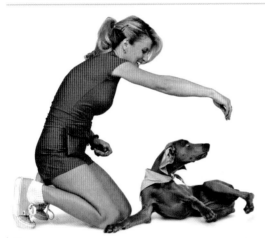

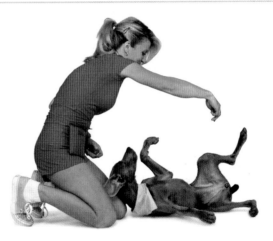

4 Cue "roll over" and make your hand signal more subtle.

Paws Up

VERBAL CUE
Paws up

"I go to Puppy Class with my owner so she can learn stuff."

Your puppy learns to put his front paws up on an object such as a box or a sturdy chair.

TEACH IT:

1 Hold a treat slightly above a sturdy box or low chair and cue your puppy "paws up." Pat the box with your other hand to coax your puppy's front paws onto it.

2 The instant both of your puppy's paws come up on the box, click your clicker, and give your puppy the treat.

3 Once your puppy gets the hang of this, try keeping your treat in your treat bag and give the cue without the food lure. If your puppy puts his paws on the box, click, and give him a treat.

WHAT TO EXPECT: Most puppies can be lured up on a box during their first training session. Some puppies are more apprehensive, and may take a second or third day.

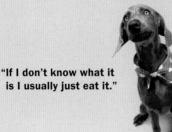

"If I don't know what it is I usually just eat it."

TROUBLESHOOTING

MY PUPPY WON'T STEP ONTO THE BOX
Encourage him by patting the box with your hand and using a happy voice. Reward just one paw on the box at first if that is all he is offering.

MY PUPPY JUMPS ON TOP OF THE BOX OR OVER THE BOX
You are holding the treat too far past the center of the box. Hold the treat only slightly beyond the far edge of the box.

TIP! Your puppy trusts you. If you tell him to step on a box, make sure the box won't fall over, as this could damage trust.

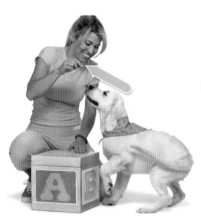

1 Use a treat to lure your puppy up. Pat the box to help coax him.

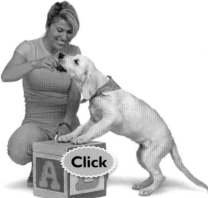

Click

2 Click once both paws are up. Allow him to have the treat.

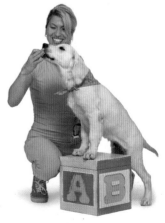

3 Next, give the cue without the food lure. Click and reward with a treat from your pocket.

Bow Your Head

Your puppy places his front paws on the edge of a bed or chair, and bows his head between his arms.

"It was an accident."

TEACH IT:

1. First, teach your puppy the **paws up** trick (page 48). Kneel in front of the box, with your puppy to your side. Hold a treat in the hand that is closest to your puppy, and hold your clicker in your other hand.

2. Use your hand with the clicker to lure your puppy to put his "paws up" on the box.

3. As soon as your puppy's paws are up, cue "prayers" and use your hand with the treat to reach up from below, luring your puppy's head down between his paws.

4. Once your puppy bows his head to follow the treat, click your clicker, and release the treat. Start by requiring only a mild bowing of his head, and be sure to give the treat only while your puppy is in the correct position—with two paws on the box and head bowed.

5. As he improves, have your puppy wait a few seconds before releasing the treat from your closed fist.

WHAT TO EXPECT: Puppies usually take a few weeks of squirming before they understand this trick.

TROUBLESHOOTING

MY PUPPY DROPS ONE PAW OFF THE BOX WHEN I OFFER THE TREAT
Offer the treat closer to his nose, and not as low. Your arm should be coming from below.

TIP! Always give the reward from below, near your puppy's chest, as rewarding from above would encourage him to peek in anticipation.

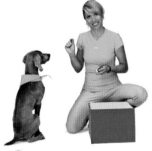

1. Hold your clicker in one hand, and a treat in the other.

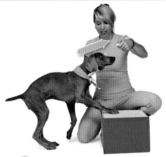

2. Use your clicker hand to lure your puppy up.

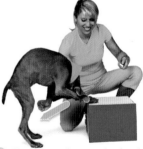

3. Use the treat in your other hand to lure your puppy's head down.

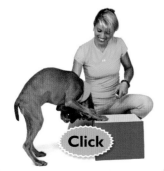

4. Click and release the treat.

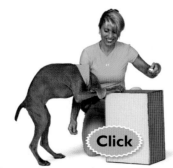

5. Have your puppy wait a few seconds before releasing the treat.

Tug

Many dogs learn to love a good game of tug with their owner, and this game can be a bonding activity as you play together.

Once you have your puppy playing tug, you can transfer that skill to teach her to pull a rope to open a door, gate, drawer, or toy box lid.

"I'm stronger then just about anybody!"

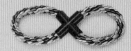

TEACH IT:

1 Choose a tug toy that is long and whippy, with fur, fleece, or leather hanging pieces. Squeakers or food pockets will be extra enticing.

2 Play with the toy; if it seems interesting to you, it will be interesting to your puppy. Slide the toy on the ground erratically away from your puppy. If your puppy is hesitant, let the toy rest on the ground for a moment and then skitter it away in fear when she approaches. Your toy should imitate a real prey animal who doesn't want to be caught.

3 Once your puppy catches the toy, say "tug" and tug the toy. Move the toy smoothly side to side (not a backward/forward tug), with an occasional careful "jerk." If the toy ever falls from your puppy's mouth, it goes back to being live prey that tries to run away. If your puppy is reluctant to tug, let go of the toy as soon as she bites it, and give her lots of praise.

4 After a few seconds of tugging, let your puppy pull the toy from your hands as her reward.

WHAT TO EXPECT: Bull breeds and terriers are naturals for this trick, but all puppies love a good pull now and then. Play daily, and within a week your puppy could tugging vigorously.

TROUBLESHOOTING

I HEARD PLAYING TUG WITH YOUR PUPPY CAUSES AGGRESSION

Tug is a prey-drive game, and it is not uncommon for puppies to growl while they are tugging. This is not necessarily aggressive behavior, but you don't want your puppy to go beyond a midlevel stimulation. If she is growling too much, end the game and put the toy away.

TIP! The more this exercise feels like a game, the faster your puppy will catch on.

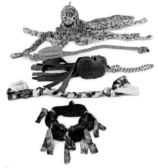

1 Choose the right tug toy for your puppy.

2 Play with the toy to get your puppy's interest.

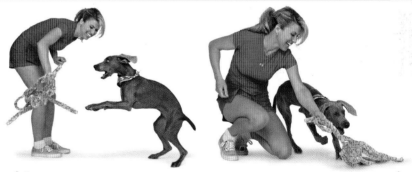

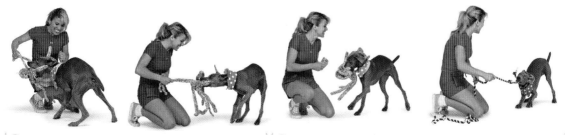

3 Play tug when your puppy catches it.

4 Let your puppy pull it from your hands.

Kisses

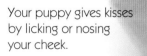

"How much longer
'til chowtime?"

Your puppy gives kisses
by licking or nosing
your cheek.

TEACH IT:

1 Sit at "puppy level" and let your puppy lick a little peanut butter off of your finger.

2 Show your puppy as you dab a little peanut butter on your cheek. Tell your puppy "kisses!"

3 As soon as your puppy touches your cheek with her nose or tongue, click your clicker and give your puppy a treat.

4 After a few repetitions of letting your puppy lick the peanut butter on your cheek, try one with no peanut butter. With a treat held behind your back, point to your cheek and tell your puppy "kisses!" When she licks or noses you, mark the instant by clicking your clicker, and then reward her with the treat from behind your back.

WHAT TO EXPECT: Puppies will often learn this trick within a week, although shy puppies may require more coaxing.

TROUBLESHOOTING

MY PUPPY BITES MY CHEEK

Puppies have sharp milk teeth, and haven't yet learned bite inhibition. Tell her "easssssy" in a drawn-out tone. If your puppy accidently bites you, say "ouch!" and move her away from you. (Be sure you stay put and move her away from you; if you were to back away from her, it could encourage her to keep coming after you in this fun game.)

TIP! Does your puppy have "puppy breath"? This is the result of blood in her mouth from teething. Give her some frozen vegetables to chew on to numb the pain.

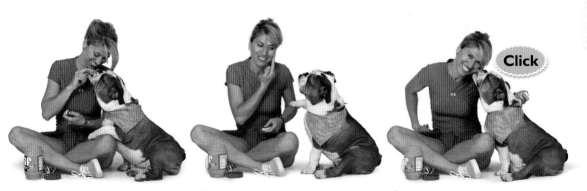

1 Let your puppy lick your finger.

2 Dab peanut butter on your cheek.

3 Click the moment your puppy touches your cheek.

Click

Head Cock

VERBAL CUE
What's that?
HAND SIGNAL

Take an adorable photo of your puppy by having him perk his ears and cock his head to the side.

"I don't like having my nails trimmed so I usually kick a lot or run away."

TEACH IT:

1 Puppies have a hard time identifying the direction of the source of a high-pitched sound, so they perk their ears and cock their head to one side to help them locate it. Select a toy that makes a long, drawn-out, high-pitched squeal. You can also use a blown-up balloon and stretch the opening into a slit, so that it squeals as the air escapes.

2 Hide the toy behind your back, and squeak it. As it is squealing, say "what's that?" in a high-pitched voice.

3 The moment you see your puppy's head cock to the side, click your clicker, and follow up with a treat.

4 Now try it without the toy. Use a high-pitched, sing-songy voice to imitate the squeal of the toy; "what's that?" Click and treat your puppy's head cock.

WHAT TO EXPECT: Some puppies cock their heads more readily than others, depending on their ear set and how they react to sound. You can often get your puppy to cock his head the first time you try.

TROUBLESHOOTING

MY PUPPY IS NOT COCKING HIS HEAD. Try different noises, such as a hiss like "psssssss," or a stacato "eee-eee-eee," or your best imitation of a creaky door opening: "creeeeak."

TIP! Puppies react most strongly to a noise the first time they hear it, and become accustomed to it over time.

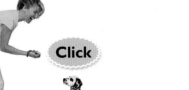

2 Hide the toy behind your back and squeak it.

3 Click and treat when your puppy cocks his head.

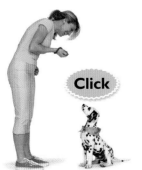

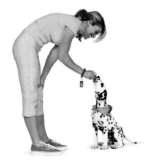

4 Use your high-pitched voice to elicit the same reaction. Click and give him a treat.

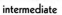

Walk on a Loose Leash

VERBAL CUE

Walkies

"I wish we could go on walks *all* the time!"

Teach your puppy to walk on a loose leash alongside you, without pulling.

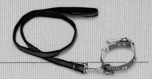

TEACH IT:

1 Take your puppy on a walk using a 6' (1.8 m) leash. Hold your leash in one hand, and your clicker in the other.

2 Any time your puppy stops pulling and lets the leash go slack, click, and give her a treat. Tell her "good walkies" so she associates positive feelings toward this word.

3 Once you've practiced several walkies using positive reinforcement rewards for polite walking, it is time to teach your puppy that there is a penalty for impolite pulling. When your puppy forges ahead and pulls on her leash, stop abruptly in your tracks. Do not allow her to pull you forward.

4 Your puppy will eventually turn around and walk toward you. When she does, click and give her a treat. Say "walkies" and start moving forward again.

WHAT TO EXPECT: In the beginning, you will find yourself stopping in your tracks very often. Don't be discouraged if it takes you ten minutes to get to the end of your driveway, as it will get easier every time. Remember to give out as many treats as penalty stops, and your puppy should be walking nicely in two to three weeks.

TROUBLESHOOTING

AM I SUPPOSED TO DO A LEASH POP WHEN SHE PULLS?

No, your intention should not be to hurt your puppy, but rather to not allow her to get what she wants by pulling. She will learn that she can move forward so long as she does so with a slack leash. Pulling will always result in a stop.

TIP! If you leave your puppy unattended, you may wish to remove her collar or use a break-away collar so that she does not get it caught on anything.

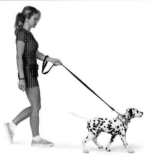

1 Hold your leash in one hand and your clicker in the other.

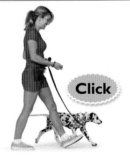 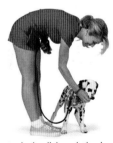

Click

2 Any time your puppy lets the leash go slack, click and give her a treat.

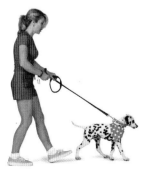

3 When your puppy pulls . . .

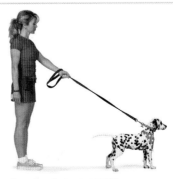

stop abruptly in your tracks.

Shake Hands

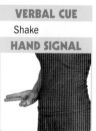

VERBAL CUE
Shake
HAND SIGNAL

"My owner says I'm going to grow up real big because I have big paws."

Teach your polite puppy to lift her paw and shake your hand. Your puppy can eventually learn to shake both her right and her left paws.

1. Hold a clicker in one hand, and in the other, hold a treat in your fist low to the ground in front of your puppy. Encourage her to paw at it by saying "get it" and "shake."

2. The moment your puppy's paw lifts off the ground, whether it touches your hand or not, click your clicker, and then open your hand and let her take the treat. Your timing of the click is very important. Try to click when her paw is off the ground, and not after she has put it back down. Be patient, as it may take several minutes to get the behavior. You can try tapping the back of your puppy's paw to give her the idea to lift it.

3. After you puppy is successful in lifting her paw, you can up the ante by challenging her to lift her paw higher. Raise the height of your hand holding the treat, and encourage your puppy to paw at it. When she does, click and open your hand to let her have the treat. Again, be sure to time the click precisely—right when her paw touches your hand.

4. Once your puppy is doing this well, it is time to try it without the treat in your hand. Hold out your empty hand and cue your puppy to "shake." When she paws at your hand, click, and then reach into your treat bag and give her a treat from there.

WHAT TO EXPECT: Some breeds are more paw-sy than others, but any puppy can learn this trick, and it's always an endearing gesture. Practice a couple of times per day, and always finish on a high note. Within two weeks your puppy could be politely proffering her paw.

TROUBLESHOOTING

INSTEAD OF PAWING AT MY HAND, MY PUPPY NOSES IT
Disregard the nosing; neither reward it nor punish it. You can move your hand out of the way when she noses it to break her train of thought. Reward any paw contact, whether or not she is nosing your hand at the same time.

TIP! Most dogs have a dominant side, so start by teaching a shake using the paw your puppy seems to prefer.

"Here're things I like: food, hot dogs, ice cubes, chasing things, biting, digging, jumping, food, furry things."

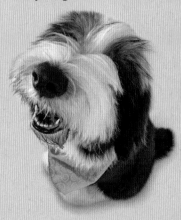

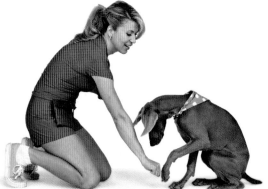

1. Hide a treat in your fist low to the ground and encourage your puppy by saying "get it! shake!"

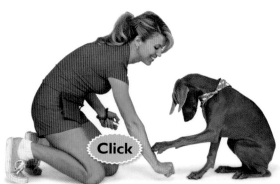

2. The moment her paw comes off the ground, click your clicker.

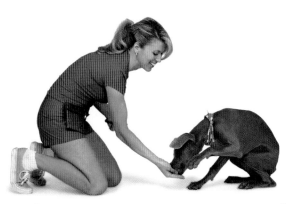

Open your hand and let your puppy have the treat.

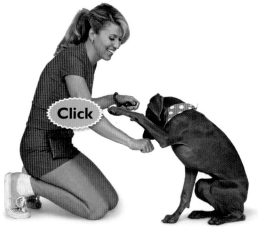

3. Raise your hand and have your puppy lift her paw higher. Click when she does.

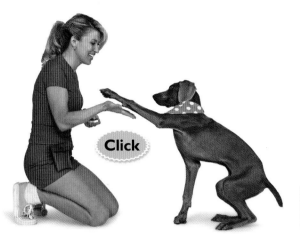

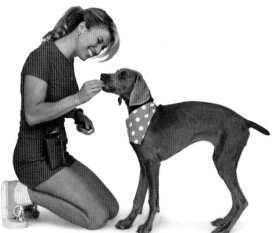

4 Hold out your empty hand and cue your puppy to "shake." Click when she paws at your hand.

Immediately take a treat from your treat bag and give her this reward.

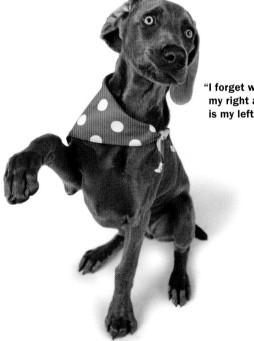

"I forget which one is my right and which one is my left."

Bark

"I like to bark! Bark, bark, bark, bark, bark!"

Teach your puppy to speak his mind by barking on your cue. Teaching your puppy a cue word for barking will also help you to communicate "no bark" when you wish him to be silent.

TEACH IT:

1 To teach this trick, you need to find a way to elicit a bark from your puppy, and then reward him for it. Puppies will often bark out of frustration. Get your puppy excited and then tease him with a treat; "Do you want it? Speak for it!" When your puppy barks, say "good bark!" and quickly give him a treat.

2 If that doesn't work, you'll have to find another stimulus that makes your puppy bark. Often a knocking sound will do the trick. Give the cue "bark," and knock on something.

3 When your puppy barks, immediately reward him, and reinforce the cue with "good bark." Repeat this process about six times.

4 Continuing in the same session, give the cue but don't knock. You may have to cue several times to get a bark. If your puppy is not barking, return to the previous steps.

WHAT TO EXPECT: Provided you've got a reliable stimulus that causes your puppy to bark, he can learn this trick in one session.

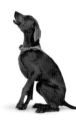

TROUBLESHOOTING

I CAN'T FIND A STIMULUS TO MAKE MY PUPPY BARK.

Try these: your doorbell, metal keys tapping on a window, or making barking sounds yourself. Play different alert sounds from your computer or phone.

TIP! Never reward your puppy for a bark unless you asked for this behavior. Otherwise he'll speak up anytime he wants something!

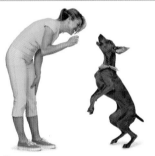

1 Tease your puppy with "Do you want it? Speak for it!"

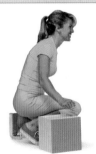

2 Cue "bark," and knock to cause your puppy to bark.

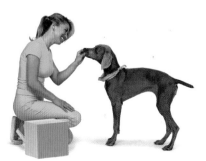

3 Immediately reward your puppy.

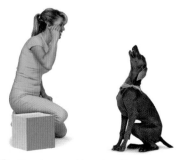

4 Give the cue without knocking.

Sing

VERBAL CUE

[howling sound]

Howling along with a dog pack is an instinctive behavior that signifies group cohesion. Even eight-week-old puppies will howl when presented with the right stimulus. If you can hit the right notes, your puppy can learn to sing along with you.

"Some of my favorite treats are cheese, cheese balls, and noodles."

TEACH IT:

1 Puppies instinctively howl along with sounds they interpret to be another howl. These are usually loud, high-pitched sounds like sirens, clarinets, and flutes. We'll use a harmonica to imitate a howl sound, as it is inexpensive and requires no musical ability on your part.

2 Stick to the higher-pitched notes on your harmonica, and blow each note for a few seconds before sliding to another note. At first, your puppy may become agitated: jumping on you, biting, pawing, or barking. This is a new experience for him, and he is deciding how to respond. Within a couple of minutes he will probably howl or whine a little.

3 Once you have your puppy singing with the harmonica, try using just your voice to elicit a howl. Keep your mouth in an oval shape, sing "ouwww" and let the howl resonate for a few seconds, gradually reducing inflection and fading out.

WHAT TO EXPECT: Northern breeds and some hounds tend to howl most readily, but all puppies have the instinct.

TROUBLESHOOTING

CAN I SKIP THE HARMONICA STEP, AND JUST USE MY VOICE?
That depends on your puppy. It is generally much easier to elicit a howl with a harmonica than with your voice.

TIP! Singing, or howling together is a bonding activity. Your puppy will enjoy this ritual with you.

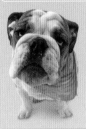

"I didn't do it."

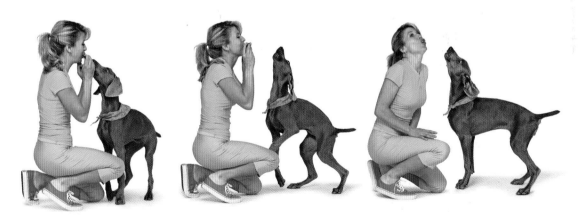

2 Your puppy may give various responses to your harmonica music.

3 Use your voice to imitate a howl, and your puppy will sing along with you.

Chapter 3:

Coordination

"I like to have stuff in my mouth and sometimes I chew it and sometimes I eat it."

Strength,

confidence, and body awareness will take time to develop in your puppy, but you can help him by training the tricks in this chapter. Your puppy will be challenged to go through a scary tunnel, balance on a wobbly teeter board, and catch a flying disk. Use lots of encouragement with your puppy, and let him approach each obstacle at his own pace. The bond that develops as you work together to achieve your goals will be worth the effort!

Some of the tricks in this chapter involve jumping. Young puppies can injure their growing bones by jumping or twisting too much. Different breeds can handle different amounts of physical stress at different ages, so you'll want to check with your veterinarian before encouraging your puppy to jump.

Make sure the ground surface has good traction, as you don't want your puppy to slip and hurt himself.

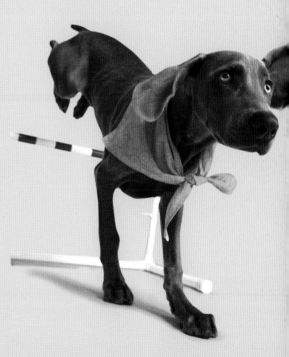

Tunnel

"Sometimes I take a shoe and then my owner chases me and it's fun."

Your puppy runs through a straight or curved tunnel. The tunnel is one of several obstacles used in the sport of dog agility. It can be a little scary the first time through, but puppies usually have great fun once they are comfortable with it!

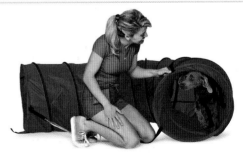

TEACH IT:

1 Allow your puppy to explore a short, straight tunnel in a familiar area. Set your puppy at the opposite end and make eye contact with her through the tunnel. Hold a treat in the tunnel and encourage her toward you by calling to her and saying "tunnel." Let her have the treat as soon as she exits.

2 Try a longer tunnel. Sit close to the entrance and toss a treat into the tunnel.

3 Once she is inside the tunnel, move to the exit, talking to your puppy the whole time so she knows where you are. Clap your hands and call to her from the exit to coax her through.

WHAT TO EXPECT: Most puppies enjoy running through a tunnel, and once accustomed to it will do so every chance they get! Confident puppies may run through the tunnel on their first day, while shy ones may require more time.

TROUBLESHOOTING

MY PUPPY DOES A U-TURN INSIDE THE TUNNEL INSTEAD OF GOING ALL THE WAY THROUGH

Toss several treats along the length of the tunnel to keep luring her forward.

MY PUPPY IS SCARED TO GO INSIDE

Don't coddle your puppy when she shows fear. Walk by the tunnel many times during the day, and your puppy will grow more confident around it.

TIP! Use sand bags inside the tunnel to keep it stationary as your puppy runs through it.

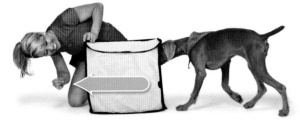

1 Coax your puppy through a short tunnel using a treat.

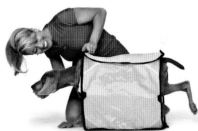

Give her the treat when she exits the tunnel.

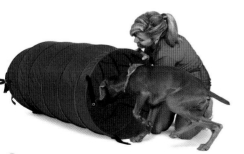

2 Toss a treat into a longer tunnel.

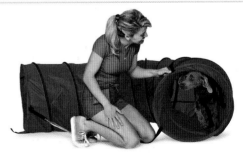

3 Call to your puppy so she knows where you are. Reward her as she exits.

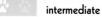
Teeter Board

The teeter-totter is an obstacle in the sport of dog agility. Young puppies can already prepare for this obstacle by learning to balance on a teeter board and becoming accustomed to the bang the board makes when it shifts.

"I have a coat that I wear when it's cold. I think it got too small though."

TEACH IT:

1 Hold your clicker in one hand, and a treat in the other. Start simply by using a treat to lure your puppy onto a plank lying on the ground. Click your clicker when he steps on it with even one paw, and let him have the treat.

2 Position a flat 2" x 4" (5 x 10 cm) board under the middle of the plank. Do not use a round dowel or triangular board, as this can cause the plank to slip when your puppy steps on it.

3 Cue "teeter" and use a treat to lure your puppy onto one end of the plank and continue to lure him forward along the plank. Don't worry if not all of his paws are on the plank.

4 When he gets to the center of the plank, his weight will pivot the plank and there will be a bang sound. The second you hear the bang, click your clicker, and let him have the treat in your hand. The bang sound can be startling for your puppy, so you want to associate it with a positive outcome (the treat).

5 Your puppy will learn that the bang of the plank is an indicator of a treat. This is a great confidence booster for your puppy, and will make his transition to the full-sized teeter-totter a cinch.

WHAT TO EXPECT: Use lots of praise and encouragement with this new and unstable obstacle, and never use force as it will heighten an already present fear. Most puppies are a little timid their first time on the teeter-totter, but conquer their fear quickly with praise and treats! Don't force the issue—tomorrow is another day and your puppy may feel differently about the obstacle then.

TROUBLESHOOTING

MY PUPPY IS AFRAID

Your puppy may be apprehensive of the wobbliness or of the banging noise. This is all the more reason to encourage your puppy to overcome his fear, and conquer this obstacle. The more you can socialize your puppy to new experiences, the more stable he will be when he grows up. The key, however, is to let him approach the feared object on his own. Encourage, but never force your puppy toward a feared object, or he may become a more fearful dog.

TIP! Dog agility is a competitive dog sport where dogs navigate through an obstacle course of teeter-totters, tire jumps, tunnels, A-frames, and more.

"I have lots and lots and lots of toys. But I probably still need a few more toys."

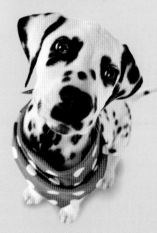

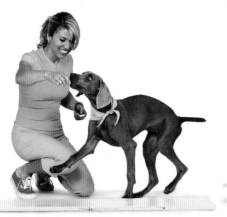

1 Lure your puppy to step onto a plank.

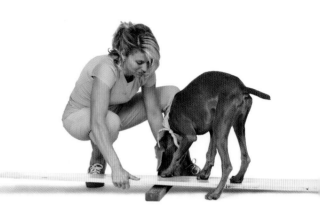

2 Position a board under the plank.

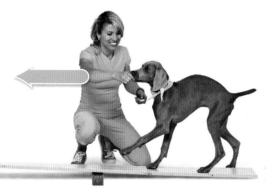

3 Lure him onto the plank with a treat.

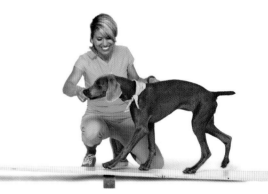

Continue to lure him across the plank.

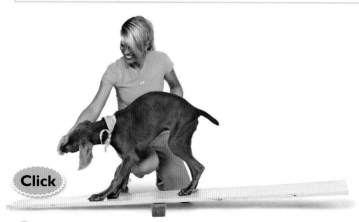

4 When the plank pivots to the other side and bangs, click, and give your puppy a treat.

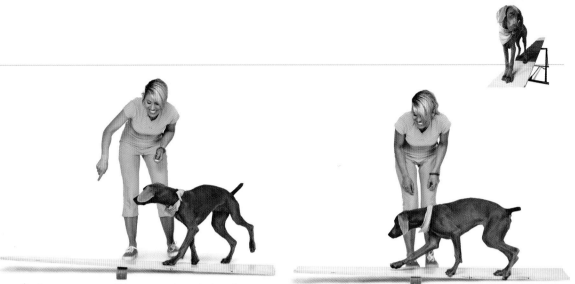

5 Soon your puppy will be eager to bang the board, as he knows the bang indicates a treat.

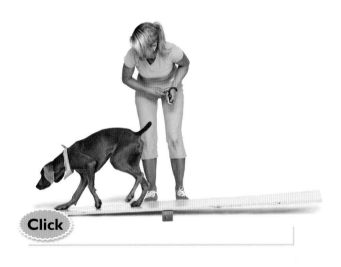

Click

"I like to make
loud noises!"

Spin

"Here're my toys: duck, frisbee, kong, bone, treat ball, tug, and squeak-squeak."

Puppies learn the spin trick quickly, and once they learn it, they will perform it every chance they get!

1. Hold a treat in your right hand, and your clicker in your left. Face your puppy and get her interested in your treat.

2. Cue your puppy to "spin," and move your right hand with the treat to your right, luring your puppy to follow.

3. Continue moving your hand forward, and all the way around in a large counterclockwise circle. Keep your hand low, at puppy-height, and move slowly so that you don't lose your puppy.

4. Once your puppy has followed your hand all the way around your circle, click your clicker, and release the treat.

5. As your puppy improves, start to trace smaller and faster circles with your treat. Eventually you will have to do no more than a flick of your wrist to your right to signal your puppy to spin. This wrist flick becomes your hand signal.

6. You can also teach your puppy to spin the the other direction. Use the same technique as spin, but cue "around" and use your left hand to trace a clockwise circle.

WHAT TO EXPECT: Practice ten times per day and in a week your puppy could be spinning circles!

TROUBLESHOOTING

MY PUPPY DOESN'T FOLLOW MY HAND
Are you using a really good treat? Try "people food" like hot dogs, chicken, or string cheese.

MY PUPPY CIRCLES IN ONE DIRECTION, BUT NOT THE OTHER
Puppies often initially have a favorite direction, but can easily become equally proficient in both directions.

MY PUPPY GOES ONLY HALFWAY
Reaching your hand too far forward too early will cause the circle to stall. Start close to your stomach and move your hand to the side before extending it forward.

TIP! Use "spin" to cue a counter-clockwise circle, and "around" to cue a clockwise circle.

"Where're you going? What're you doing? Why'd you do that? What's that? What're you doing now?"

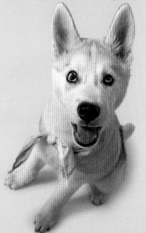

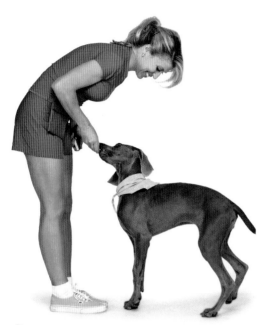

1 Face your puppy and get her interested in your treat.

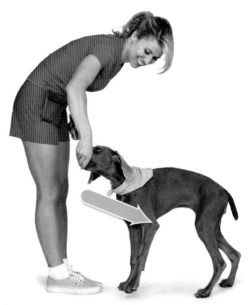

2 Move your right hand to your right . . .

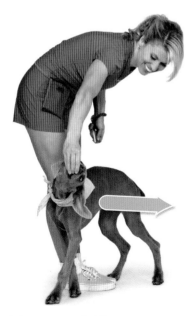

luring your puppy to follow.

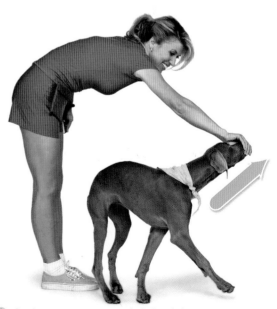

3 Continue to trace a counterclockwise circle.

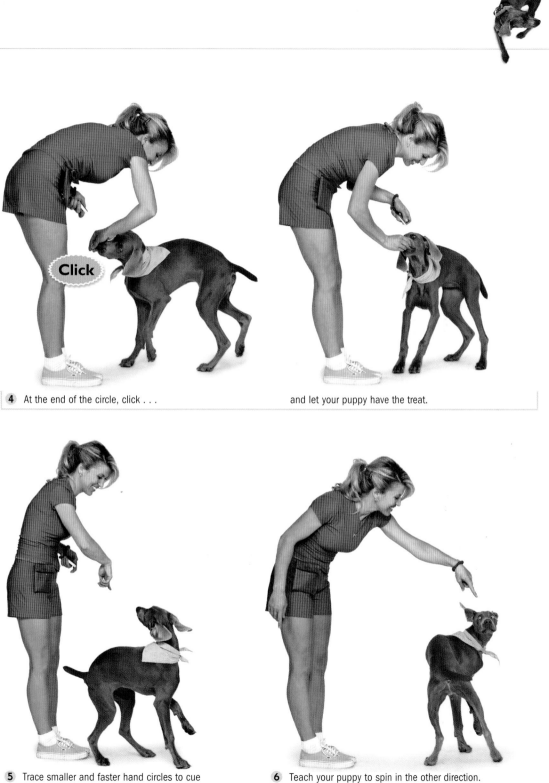

4 At the end of the circle, click . . .

Click

and let your puppy have the treat.

5 Trace smaller and faster hand circles to cue your puppy.

6 Teach your puppy to spin in the other direction.

Figure-8s

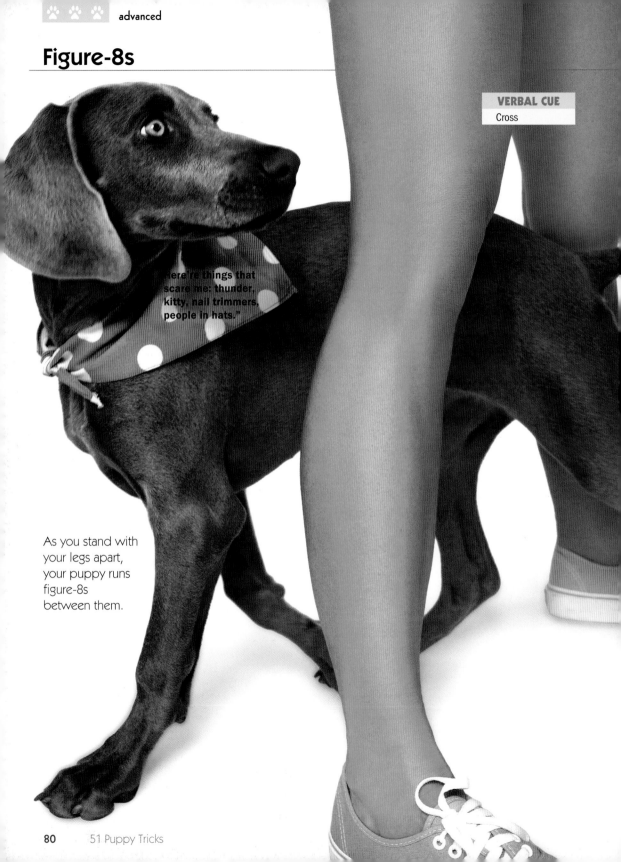

"Here're things that scare me: thunder, kitty, nail trimmers, people in hats."

As you stand with your legs apart, your puppy runs figure-8s between them.

1. Start by holding several small treats in each of your hands. Stand with your legs apart, and your puppy on your left side. Get your puppy's attention with the treat in your left hand.

2. Cue "cross" and move your treat at your puppy's nose height, forward, and between your legs. Think of your treat as an imaginary leash to "pull" your puppy through your legs from front to back.

3. At the point where your left hand is between your legs, reach your right hand behind your leg to meet your left hand. Pull your left hand away, and continue to lure your puppy with your right hand.

4. Once you have lured your puppy through your legs, continue to move your right hand forward, luring your puppy to your right side. When your puppy's head is alongside your right leg, let her have one of the treats from your right hand. Be sure to give the treat when your puppy is in this position, at the side of your leg, as this is the position where your puppy is the most apt to continue moving forward.

5. Since you started with several treats in each hand, you should still have another treat in your right hand which you can use to continue to lure your puppy forward and between your legs. Again, meet your hands together between your legs. Withdraw your right hand, and continue luring with your left hand. Reward your puppy when she is alongside your left leg.

6. As your puppy improves, use your pointed finger to lure your puppy around your legs rather than the food lure. Keep your feet planted but lunge to each side as your puppy crosses between your legs. As she crosses between your legs in preparation for circling your right leg, your right leg should be bent, and she should see your right hand guiding her through your legs and toward your right leg. Have your puppy do several figure-8's before giving her a treat, but continue the habit of only rewarding alongside your leg. Reward sometimes alongside your left leg and sometimes alongside your right, so your puppy does each side with equal eagerness.

7. Finally, stand up straight and just use a pointed finger along your side and say "cross" to cue your puppy.

WHAT TO EXPECT: A puppy can be following your food lure through your legs in a few days. In two or three weeks she can be jogging easily through your legs.

TROUBLESHOOTING

I'M HAVING TROUBLE GETTING MY PUPPY TO FOLLOW MY FOOD LURE

Some puppies are either not that interested in a food lure, or so hyper that they are not following the lure smoothly. For these puppies, you can attach a tab lead—a short, 12" (30.5 cm) leash—and guide them through that way.

TIP! Make sure your puppy always passes through your legs approaching from your front. This allows you to watch her approach.

"Can I have a cookie? I'll be really, really good. I promise."

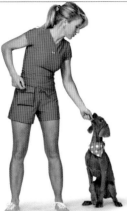 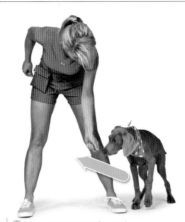 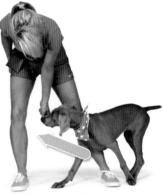

1 Start with your puppy on your left.　2 Lure your puppy forward . . .　and between your legs.

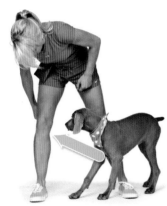 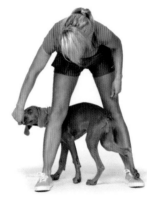

3 Switch hands and lure your puppy with your right hand.　4 Let her have the treat at the side of your leg.

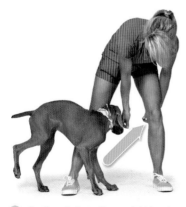 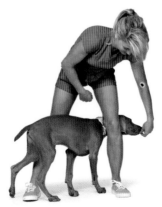 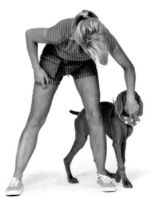

5 Continue luring with your right hand, and bring your left hand to meet it.　Now lure with your left hand.　Reward alongside your leg.

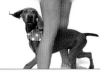

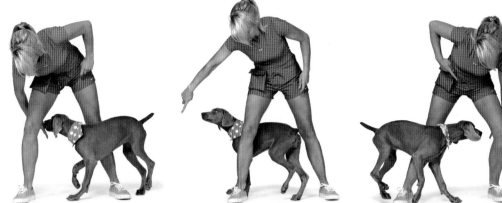

6 Use your pointed finger and lunge to each side as your puppy pass through.

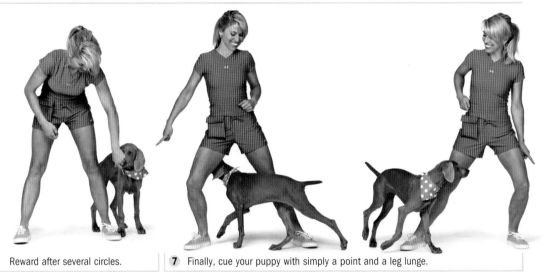

Reward after several circles.

7 Finally, cue your puppy with simply a point and a leg lunge.

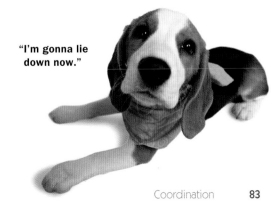

"I'm gonna lie down now."

Volleyball

Toss a lightweight ball or a balloon to your puppy, and teach him to bounce it back to you using his nose. This trick will help your puppy develop motor function and coordination skills.

"Sometimes we visit the vet and he has a furry mustache and sometimes he lets me chew on it."

TEACH IT:

1 The first step to teaching volleyball is to teach your puppy to catch a tossed item. Use a soft plush toy, and get your puppy interested in it by squiggling it around and squeaking it if it has a squeaker.

2 When your puppy is focused on the toy, say "catch!" and toss it up in a slow arc toward your puppy. Use your clicker to mark the instant he catches the toy, and then follow up with a treat.

3 Once your puppy is pretty good at catching a toy, switch to a large lightweight ball or a balloon (a regulation volleyball is too heavy for your puppy). Face your puppy and cue "bounce" as you toss the ball in a high arc so that it will come down rather vertically above your puppy's nose. Because of the large circumference of the ball, your puppy will be unable to catch it, and the ball will instead bounce off his nose and in a similar high arc back to you. Yay, you did it!

WHAT TO EXPECT: This trick is often easier to teach than it looks! Once your puppy is able to catch a toy, he could be bouncing a toy volleyball off his nose in his first training session!

TROUBLESHOOTING

MY PUPPY IS SCARED OF THE FALLING BALL

Don't toss the ball *at* your puppy, but rather in an arc that falls down right in front of your puppy. You can also try using a balloon, as it falls more slowly through the air.

TIP! If you use a balloon for this trick, clean up the pieces if the balloon pops so that your puppy does not eat them.

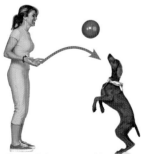

1 Get your puppy interested in a plush toy.

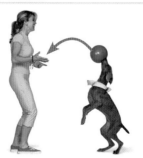

2 Toss the toy to your puppy, and click his catch.

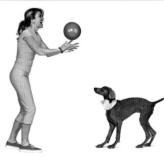

Follow up with a treat.

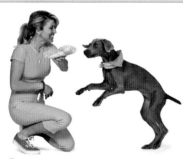

3 Toss a lightweight ball in a high arc and cue "bounce."

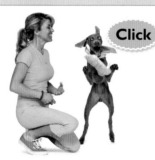

When you puppy tries to catch it, it will bounce off his nose.

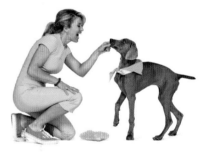

Yay! You did it!

Jump Over My Leg

As you kneel on the floor, your puppy jumps over your extended leg. Your puppy can learn to run circles around you, jumping your leg each time.

"Sometimes I jump on my owner's bed in the morning because she sleeps too much and I need to wake her up."

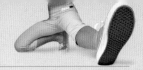

TEACH IT:

1. Kneel on the ground with your right leg outstretched. Placing your toe against a wall will prevent your puppy from going around your leg. Hold your clicker in your left hand and a treat in your right. Start with your puppy on your left side, and lure him over your leg with the treat. An enthusiastic "hup!" will stimulate him into action! If your puppy is reluctant, lure him slowly so that he first places his front paws on your thigh. Allow him to nibble the treat from this position, then move the treat farther away. Your puppy may be tempted to cross near your ankle as that is the lowest spot, so keep your treat close to your body to tempt him in that direction. As he crosses over your leg, click your clicker, and then let him have the treat.

2. Start with your puppy on your left. This time, switch hands so that your clicker is in your right hand and a treat is in your left. Use your clicker as a lure to guide your puppy's attention over your leg. Click as your puppy is jumping or walking over your leg.

3. Use your right hand to guide your puppy's attention around toward your back. Move your left hand to meet your right hand behind your back. Wiggle the treat in your left hand to get your puppy to focus on it instead of your clicker, and move your clicker hand out of the way. Using the treat in your left hand, continue to guide your puppy around your back, and to your left side.

4. Once your puppy has made it all the way around your body back to your left side, let him have the treat. In this trick the treat will always be given at your left side, as this will encourage a speedy jump and circle from your puppy.

5. After giving your treat, immediately refocus your puppy on the clicker in your right hand, and guide him over your leg again to repeat the whole routine.

6. Once your puppy has the hang of this, put away your clicker and instead use a pointed finger and a sweeping motion of your right arm to signal your puppy to jump over your leg. As always, reward your puppy at your left side.

WHAT TO EXPECT: This is usually a fun trick for puppies, and one that they enjoy performing. Practice when your puppy is full of energy and he should get the hang of it within a week!

TROUBLESHOOTING

I'M NOT PHYSICALLY ABLE TO KNEEL IN THIS POSITION

Try this variation: Sit in a chair facing a wall. Extend both of your feet, with your toes on the floor, touching the base of the wall. Lean forward in your chair and lure your puppy over your legs. Instead of having your puppy circle behind you, hold treats in both hands and have him jump back and forth over your legs.

TIP! Don't encourage your puppy to jump high, as it could injure his growing bones.

"Once I found a big toad and he jumped and I was scared of him at first but then I wasn't scared any more."

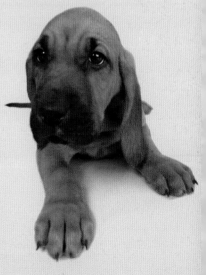

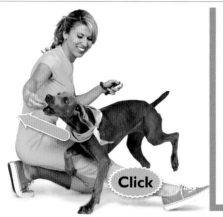

1. Put your right foot against the wall. Lure your puppy over your leg with a treat. Click as he passes over your leg.

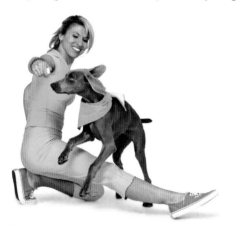

2. Switch your clicker into your right hand and a treat into your left. Guide your puppy with your clicker hand.

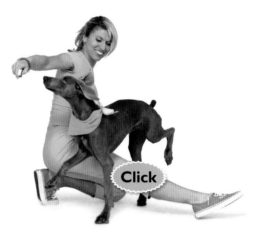

Click when your puppy crosses over your leg.

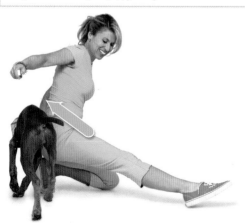

3. Connect your hands behind your back and refocus his attention on the treat in your left hand.

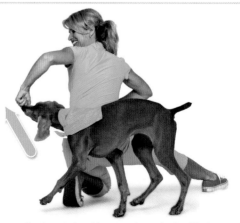

Continue to lure him around your body with the treat in your left hand.

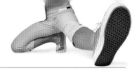

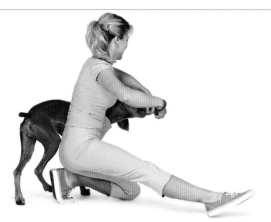

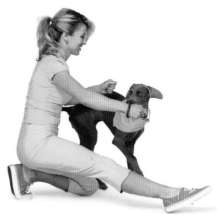

4 Once your puppy has made it around to your left side, let him have the treat.

5 Refocus your puppy's attention on the clicker in your right hand and repeat the process.

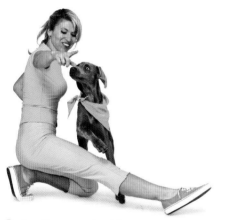

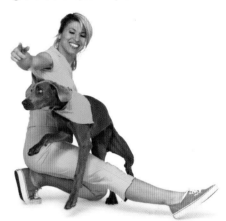

6 Transition to a pointed finger.

Use a sweeping motion of your right arm to signal your puppy.

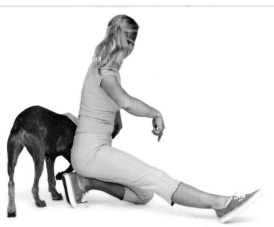

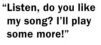

Always reward your puppy when he comes around to your left side.

"Listen, do you like my song? I'll play some more!"

Hoop Jump

Hup

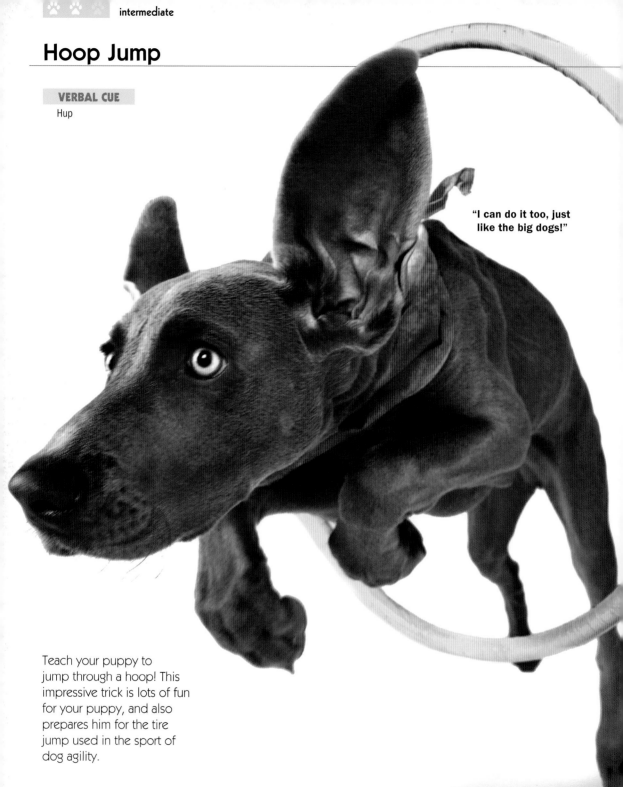

"I can do it too, just like the big dogs!"

Teach your puppy to jump through a hoop! This impressive trick is lots of fun for your puppy, and also prepares him for the tire jump used in the sport of dog agility.

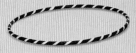

1. Remove the noisy beads within a toy hula hoop as they may frighten your puppy. Allow her time to investigate the hoop and overcome any fear she has of it. Puppies can be frightened to go through the hoop for the first time, and it is important that you allow your puppy to make the decision to go through on her own, without forcing her.

2. Hold your hoop across a doorway, with your puppy on one side of the doorway, and you on the other. Use the hand that is closest to your puppy to hold both the hoop and also your clicker. Hold a treat in your other hand, and use it to lure your puppy through the hoop. Click the moment she crosses through the hoop and allow her to take the treat on the other side.

3. Now try it in an open room. Hold the hoop on the ground with the hand closest to your puppy, tell her "hup," and lure her through with a treat in your other hand. Click when she goes through, and let her have the treat on the other side.

4. As your puppy gets the idea, begin to raise the hoop off the floor. Depending on a puppy's age, she should be jumping no higher than her ankle, knee, or chest height (consult with your veterinarian for specifics.) Puppies sometimes get tangled in the hoop, so be prepared to release it if you feel resistance. Use your hand opposite your puppy to lure her energetically upward.

WHAT TO EXPECT: Puppies usually get the hang of hoop jumping within a weeks or two and do it enthusiastically.

TROUBLESHOOTING

THE HOOP FELL ON MY PUPPY AND NOW SHE IS FRIGHTENED OF IT!
Puppies pick up on your energy. Don't coddle your puppy; just act like it is not a big deal and proceed with the lesson.

TIP! Challenging your puppy early with varied obstacles will make her a more confident dog.

"I did good today!"

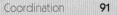

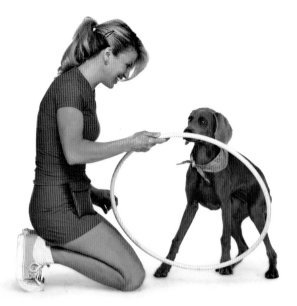

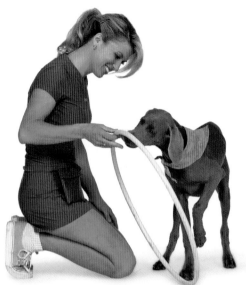

1 Puppies may be initially fearful of the hoop . . .

Allow your puppy time to investigate the hoop, and overcome her fears.

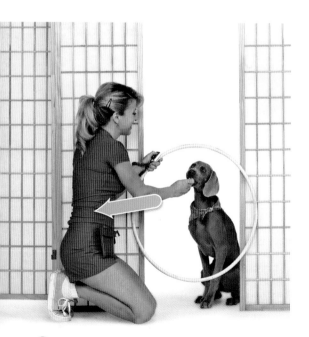

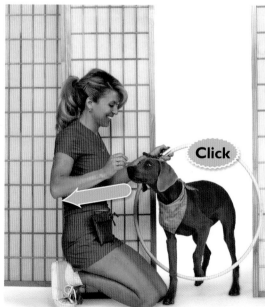

Click

2 Use the hand that is closest to your puppy to hold both the hoop and your clicker.

Lure your puppy through the hoop with your other hand. Click as she goes through the hoop.

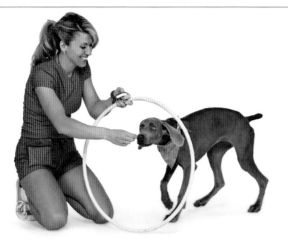

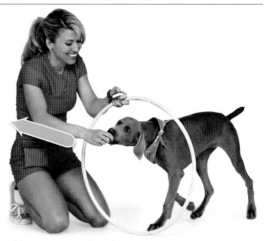

3 Place the hoop on the ground . . .

and lure your puppy through.

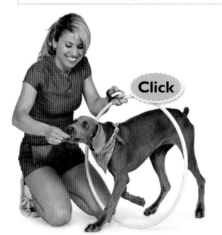

Click when she crosses through the hoop . . .

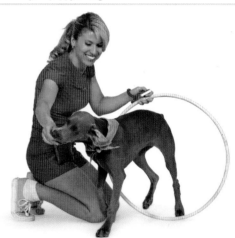

and allow her to have the treat.

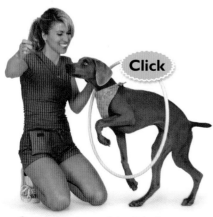

4 Raise the hoop a little off the floor.

"I was playing with my ball but then it got lost and I can't find it!"

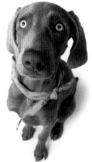

Hide Yourself in a Box

In this adorable trick, your puppy learns to jump inside a box to "hide" himself.

"I chased a puppy at the park but then he chased me so I ran away."

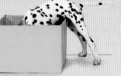

TEACH IT:

1 Show your puppy a treat, and toss it inside a box. Tilt the box up, so your puppy can reach in and get the treat.

2 Toss in another treat. Tilt the box up so your puppy can see the treat, but then lay it flat again. Allow your puppy time to experiment and decide what to do. If he loses interest, tilt the box up again, showing him the treat. A confident puppy will eventually put his front paws in the box in order to get the treat. Click your clicker when he does this, and allow him to eat the treat.

3 This time, instead of tossing the treat inside the box, say "go hide" and, holding the treat in your hand, use it to lure your puppy to step into the box. Stand opposite your puppy, with the box between you. Get your puppy's interest by showing him the treat in front of his nose. Move the treat away from him and over the box. As soon as his front paws are in the box, click your clicker, and give him the treat.

4 Continue to lure your puppy farther into the box by positioning another treat just out of his reach. As soon as all four paws make it inside the box, click, and give him the treat.

WHAT TO EXPECT: Your puppy's success with this trick will depend a lot on the type of box you choose. A large, shallow box will be easiest to start, and you can work your way up to smaller and higher boxes.

TROUBLESHOOTING

I CAN'T LURE MY PUPPY INTO THE BOX. CAN I PICK HIM UP AND PUT HIM IN THERE?

Puppies will develop much more confidence if they are allowed to approach an item on their own terms, rather than being forced into it. It may take longer to teach it this way, but by encouraging— rather than forcing— your puppy into the box, you are putting him on the path to becoming a more confident adult dog.

TIP! Expose your puppy to all sorts of obstacles; boxes, teeter boards, slippery surfaces, water. This early exposure will make him a more confident dog.

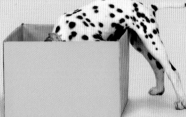

"I like to get in my box! And then I like to jump out of my box!"

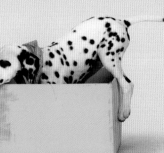

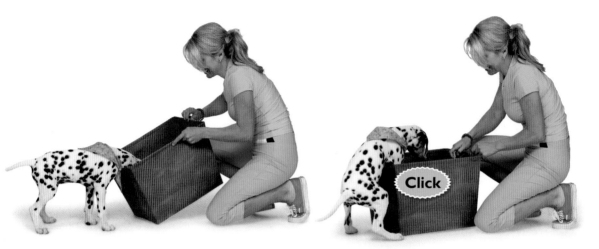

1 Tilt the box so your puppy can take the treat.

2 Let your puppy figure out how to put his front paws inside the box. Click when he does.

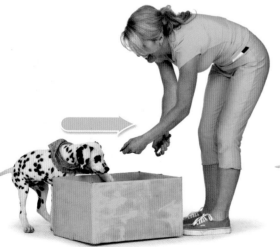

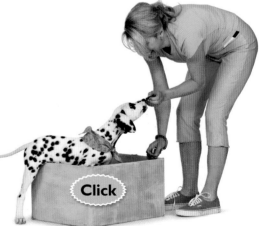

3 Lure him into the box by moving a treat from his nose toward the center of the box.

When he puts his paws in the box, click, and give him the treat.

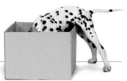

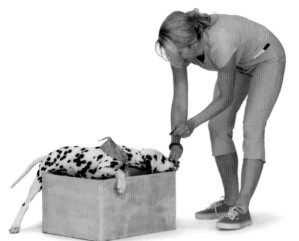

4 Continue to lure him farther into the box with another treat.

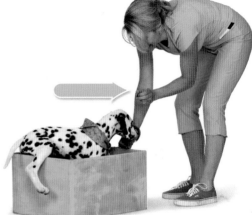

Hold the treat just out of his reach.

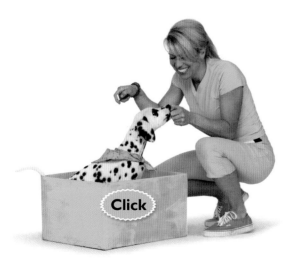

Click

When all four paws are in the box, click, and treat.

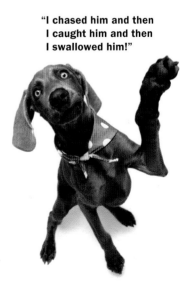

"I chased him and then I caught him and then I swallowed him!"

Wipe Your Paws

"I can dig really big holes!"

Your polite puppy can learn to scratch her front paws on a doormat. Say good-bye to muddy pawprints on your floor!

TEACH IT:

1 Let your puppy watch as you place a treat under the corner of a doormat.

2 Encourage your puppy to go after the treat by saying "dig! Get it! Get it!" and tapping the doormat. If your puppy loses interest, quickly lift the corner of the doormat to reveal the treat again. If your puppy tries to use her nose to poke under the doormat, hold the doormat down with your hand. Within about a minute, your puppy will probably scratch at the doormat—be ready! The instant she scratches even once, click your clicker.

3 Immediately after your click, lift the corner of the doormat and let her have the treat.

4 As your puppy improves, wait for her to do two or three scratches before you click and lift the doormat.

WHAT TO EXPECT: Puppies can have some success with this trick on their first day. Eventually your puppy will do this trick on cue, and you won't need to hide the treat any more. Instead, after a few scratches, toss the treat on top of the doormat, so your puppy still has the excitement of finding her treasure.

TROUBLESHOOTING

MY PUPPY WON'T SCRATCH THE DOORMAT

Try another tactic: Take a favorite ball or toy, and hide it in sand or loose dirt. The second your puppy scratches for it, click and treat. Once she understands this cue, you can transfer the behavior to the doormat.

TIP! Use hard treats when teaching this trick, as soft treats tend to squish and make a mess!

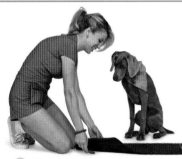

1 Place a treat under the doormat.

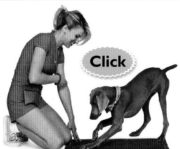

2 Click when your puppy does a single scratch.

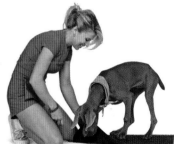

3 Lift the doormat to let her have the treat.

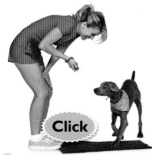

4 Wait for her to do two or three scratches before you click.

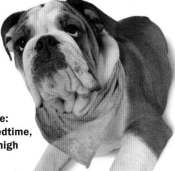

"Here're things I don't like: dogs that bark at me, bedtime, when my owner leaves, high kitchen counters."

Flying Disc

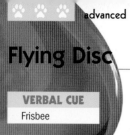

VERBAL CUE
Frisbee

"One time I caught
a bird right out of
the sky! Well, it was
a flying disc, but it
could've been a bird."

Learning to catch a flying
disc will help your puppy
build coordination and will
become a great way
to exercise your dog
throughout her life.

TEACH IT:

1 Hard plastic toy discs could injure your puppy's mouth and teeth. Use only discs specifically designed for a dog, such as a soft plastic, flexible rubber, or canvas disc. Introduce your puppy to this fun new toy by tossing it playfully, playing keep away and tug with it.

2 Get your puppy's interest by spinning the upside-down disc in circles.

3 When she shows interest, throw a "roller"—rolling the disc along its edge. Encourage your puppy excitedly to "Get it! Get it!" and praise her heavily when she does.

4 Teach your puppy to catch the disc in midair by throwing it in a low, flat trajectory. Do not throw it directly at your puppy, as you don't want to hit her with it.

WHAT TO EXPECT: It could take months for your puppy to build the coordination to master an airborne catch. Keep the game fun, and work in short sessions. Puppies under fourteen months should not be jumping for the disc, and all puppies should be checked by a veterinarian to ensure soundness.

TROUBLESHOOTING

MY PUPPY IS NOT INTERESTED IN THE DISC

Increase the value of this toy by turning it upside down and using it as your puppy's feeding dish. She will come to associate the sight and smell of it with her dinner.

TIP! Specially fabricated plastic dog discs are soft enough to be easily scratched with your fingernail.

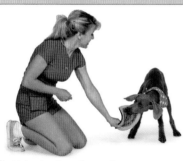

1 Make the disc a fun toy for your puppy.

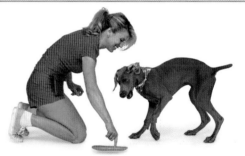

2 Spin the disc in circles.

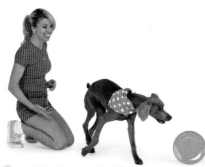

3 Roll the disc along its side.

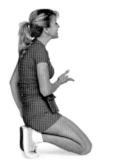

4 Toss the disc in the air for your puppy to catch.

Chapter 4:

Communication

"Pay attention to me;
pay attention to me;
pay attention to me!"

Listening

to your puppy is just as important as talking to your puppy. Show your puppy that she can depend on you to take care of her by being responsive to her needs and wishes.

In this chapter are tricks that will enhance human-puppy communication. Some tricks teach your puppy appropriate ways to convey her wishes, such as by ringing a bell on the doorknob when she needs to go potty, or bringing her leash when she wants a walk.

Other tricks in this chapter teach your puppy to play a game with you, such as "Which Hand Holds the Treat?" And other tricks begin to teach your puppy basic house manners, such as "Sit before Chowtime."

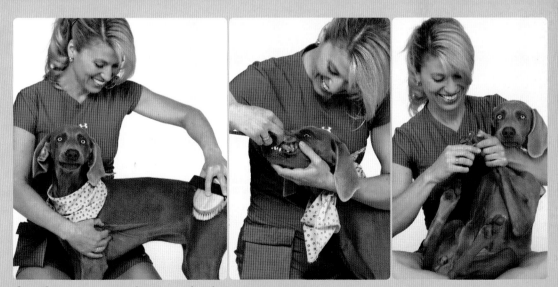

Care for your puppy by grooming her.

Ring a Bell to Go Outside

Your puppy rings a bell on the door to let you know that she needs to go outside. This trick can be taught to young puppies who are being house-trained.

"I hafta go potty now."

TEACH IT:

1 Hang a bell from a doorknob at a low height. Dab a little peanut butter on the inside of the bell and encourage your puppy to explore it by wiggling it and saying "bell, get it!" The instant your puppy causes the bell to ring, click your clicker and give her a treat from your hand.

2 Don't replenish the peanut butter, as there is probably a trace amount still on the bell. Point to the bell again, and click and treat again when your puppy rings it. Repeat this process several times. If your puppy seems confused, go back to using the peanut butter.

3 Get your puppy's leash and get her excited to go for a walk. Stop at the door with the bell, encouraging her to ring it. It may take a while, but as soon as she touches the bell, immediately open the door and take her outside. In this trick, the reward is access to the outdoors instead of a treat, so be sure to introduce this concept early on.

WHAT TO EXPECT: The more responsive you are to the bells in the beginning, the quicker your puppy will learn this trick. Most puppies will start ringing the bell on their own within a week.

TROUBLESHOOTING

WHEN I CLICK MY PUPPY FOR LICKING THE PEANUT BUTTER, SHE DOESN'T TAKE THE TREAT FROM MY HAND, BUT JUST KEEPS LICKING THE PEANUT BUTTER

The important thing is that you *offer* the treat. It is not critical that your puppy takes it. You can also try using a really good treat, like steak, chicken, or cheese.

TIP! Use a large bell, rather than small jingle bells that could be swallowed by a puppy.

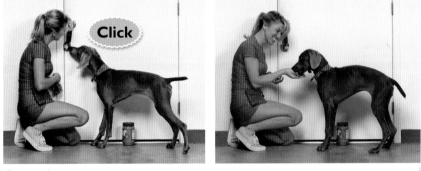

1 Dab peanut butter on the bell and reward your puppy for making it ring.

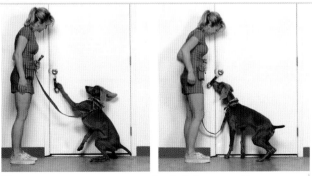

3 Before a walk, have your puppy ring the bell to go outside.

"I like to make noise!"

Get Your Leash

"Sometimes I get scared of the mean dog down the street and I run behind my owner's legs."

Teach your puppy to fetch his leash when it's time for a walk.

TEACH IT:

1 You'll want to first teach your puppy how to **fetch** (page 134). Introduce the word "leash" to your puppy by using it each time you put it on him. Fasten his leash together in a bundle with a rubber band and toss it playfully. Tell him to "fetch leash" and give him a treat when he returns.

2 Now put the leash in its regular spot, such as on a table by the door. Point to it and encourage your puppy to "get your leash!"

3 Reward your puppy by immediately attaching his leash to his collar and taking him out for a walk. In this trick, the reward is a walk instead of a treat, so be sure to introduce this concept early on.

WHAT TO EXPECT: Don't be surprised if your puppy communicates his wishes to you by dropping his leash in your lap! Try to reward his politeness with a walk as often as possible.

TROUBLESHOOTING

DO I HAVE TO TEACH "FETCH" BEFORE I TEACH THIS TRICK?

If you haven't already taught your puppy to fetch, try this: Bundle the leash in a bunch, and toss it playfully. As soon as your puppy puts his mouth on it, click your clicker, give him a treat, and then take him immediately for a walk.

TIP! The next time you are ready to go for a walk, get your puppy excited to go out, and then have him get his leash before leaving.

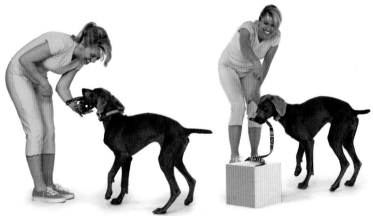

1 Toss the leash and have your puppy "fetch."

2 Put the leash in its regular spot.

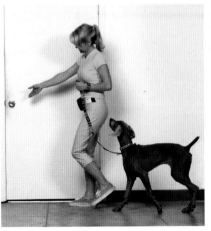

3 Reward your puppy by attaching his leash and taking him for a walk.

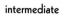
Bring Your Food Dish

"I think it's time to eat now."

Having your puppy fetch bowl before receiving his dinner teaches him about working to receive rewards. Plus, it's just darn cute!

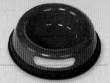

TEACH IT:

1 First, teach your puppy to **fetch** (page 134) and **fetch to hand** (page 138).

2 Start your routine of preparing your puppy's dinner . . . go to the kitchen, get out the bag of dog food, etc.

3 Point to your puppy's bowl and tell him to "fetch!" He will likely be excited and spinning circles, and forget what he's doing. Keep pointing to the bowl and encouraging him.

4 When he finally brings his bowl to you, praise him excitedly. Immediately put his dinner or some treats in the bowl, lower it to the ground, and let him eat his reward.

WHAT TO EXPECT: The challenge in teaching this trick will be in the first time you train it. Once your puppy has one success, he will very quickly make the association between bringing his bowl and getting his dinner.

TROUBLESHOOTING

MY PUPPY WILL FETCH OTHER THINGS, BUT NOT HIS FOOD DISH
The problem may be the specific food dish. Puppies are reluctant to put metal or porcelain in their mouths, so use a plastic bowl. Make sure the bowl has a lip, groove, or other feature that will allow your puppy to easily grasp it.

TIP! Puppies should be fed three meals per day until they are about five months old. After that, they need two meals per day.

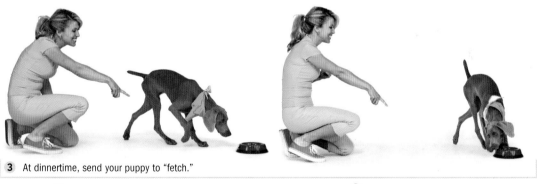

3 At dinnertime, send your puppy to "fetch."

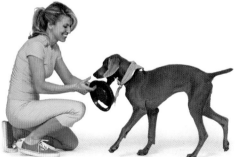

4 Praise him when he returns with his bowl . . .

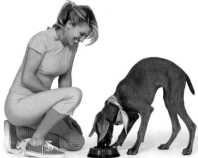

and immediately feed him his dinner.

Sit before Chowtime

"My owner says we
have manners in
this house."

It's never too early to start learning
manners. Teach your polite puppy to
sit before her dinner is served.

TEACH IT:

1 First teach your puppy to **sit** (page 38). When it is meal time, prepare your puppy's bowl and hold it out of her reach. Tell her to "chowtime, sit." Because she is a puppy, she will be so excited that she may temporarily have forgotten the meaning of the word! Give her several chances to sit, and help her by using the food bowl to lure her head up and back, causing her rear to drop. If she does not sit, turn away and put the bowl out of her reach for a minute.

2 Try again a minute later. When your puppy does finally sit, even for a second, mark that instant my saying "good" or clicking your clicker.

3 Immediately put her bowl down as a reward for her politeness.

WHAT TO EXPECT: Puppies as young as eight weeks are capable of learning to sit before chowtime. This exercise helps build good manners in your puppy. Don't be too strict with your puppy, as the goal is not that she do a perfect sit, but rather that she build a habit of asking politely for her dinner rather than demanding it.

TROUBLESHOOTING

MY PUPPY JUST WON'T SIT

It's not fair to ask your puppy to sit before chowtime if she hasn't been taught to sit in the first place, so give some thought as to whether that may be the problem. If she has been taught to sit, then try holding the food bowl above her head and moving toward her. This should cause her rear to drop, especially if her back is against a wall.

TIP! Don't "free feed" your puppy. Instead, offer her a meal, and if she hasn't finished it in fifteen minutes, pick up the bowl.

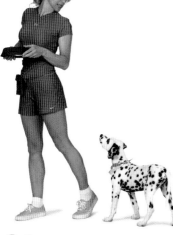

1 If your puppy does not sit, put the bowl away for a minute.

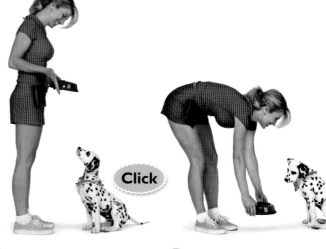

2 Mark the instant your puppy sits.

3 Immediately give her the food.

Leave It

VERBAL CUE

Leave it

"Once I found a
sandwich on the
table. I look there
all the time but
I haven't found
another one yet."

When you don't want your
puppy to eat something—
or to even approach
something— tell him to
"leave it." This command
can apply to a doughnut,
your shoe, or your cat.

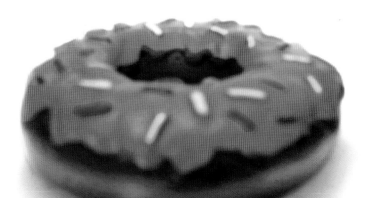

1. Sit with your puppy and place a treat on the ground. In an authoritative (but not loud) voice, tell him to "leave it." Keep your hand ready to cover the treat if he goes for it.

2. When he shows interest in the treat, tell him "no" and cover the treat with your hand.

3. Repeat this process until your puppy refrains from moving toward the treat. At first, he may only refrain for a second or two before he changes his mind and goes for the treat. You want to reward your puppy before he changes his mind. Study how long it takes him to break, and reward him a second before he breaks. Click your clicker and hand him a treat from your pocket.

WHAT TO EXPECT: Most puppies can learn this trick within a week. Always reward your puppy with a treat from your hand, rather than allowing him to take the treat from the floor, as allowing him to take the treat from the floor would teach him to fixate on that item. You instead want him to ignore the item.

TROUBLESHOOTING

MY PUPPY NEVER STOPS GOING FOR THE TREAT!

Patience . . . if you block him enough times from getting the treat, he will eventually pause. Click that small pause and reward him! Timing is crucial; be sure to click while he is paused, and not after he has moved toward the treat.

TIP! You can also use "leave it" to keep your puppy from approaching your shoe, your cat, or anything else he is to stay away from.

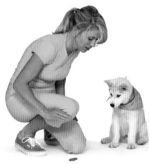

1. Tell your puppy to "leave it."

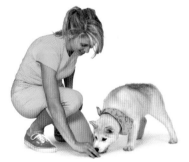

2. When your puppy approaches the treat, cover it up.

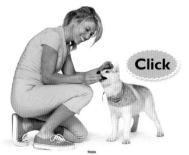

3. Click and reward your puppy when he refrains from moving toward the treat.

"Youuuu can't catch meeeee!"

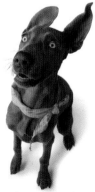

Which Hand Holds the Treat?

VERBAL CUE
Which hand?

HAND SIGNAL

VERBAL CUE
Which hand?

HAND SIGNAL

"This is my best trick!"

When presented with your two closed fists, your puppy sniffs each and indicates which hand holds the treat.

TEACH IT:

1. Hold a strong-smelling treat slightly exposed in one of your two fists. Present your fists at your puppy's chest height and ask him "which hand?"

2. When your puppy shows interest in the correct hand by nosing or pawing it, mark that instant by saying "good!" and open your hand to allow him to take the treat.

3. If your puppy shows interest in the wrong hand, tell him "whoops;" open that hand to show him it is empty. Wait ten seconds before trying again so that there are negative consequences to his incorrect choice.

4. Once your puppy is consistently nosing your correct hand, try to get him to paw at your correct hand instead. Keep your fists low to the ground. When your puppy has indicated his choice with his nose, pull your other hand back and encourage him to paw at your correct hand by saying "get it!"

WHAT TO EXPECT: This trick is usually a favorite, as it involves two of your puppy's favorite things: using his nose and getting treats!

TROUBLESHOOTING

I THINK MY PUPPY IS JUST GUESSING

Overly zealous puppies will be in such a hurry to get the treat that they paw at the first hand they see. Try holding your fists up above your puppy's head so he can sniff them but not paw them. After he has sniffed both, tell him to "wait," lower your hands, and then ask "which hand?"

TIP! Microwave hot dog slices on a paper towel–covered plate three minutes for a tasty training treat!

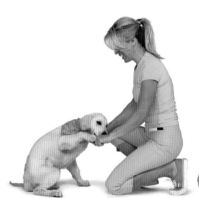

2. When your puppy shows interest in the correct hand, say "good" and open your hand.

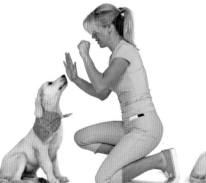

3. If your puppy chooses the wrong hand, say "whoops!"

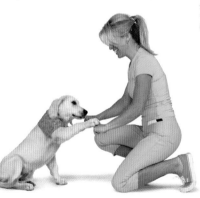

4. See if you can get your puppy to indicate his choice with his paw.

Shell Game

VERBAL CUE
Find it

In the classic game, a ball is placed beneath one of three pails, or shells. The shells are quickly shuffled, and your puppy shows you which one is hiding the ball.

"My owner said she should have named me Trouble, but I like Jadie better."

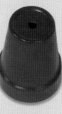

1. You'll need three identical flower pots for this trick. The pots should have a hole at the base, which will allow your puppy to smell the treat hidden under it. Heavy clay flower pots will work best because they won't overturn easily when your puppy sniffs them. Start with just one flower pot and rub the inside with an aromatic treat (such as hot dog, steak, or chicken) to give it lots of scent. Let your puppy watch as you place a treat on the floor and cover it with the pot.

2. Encourage him to "find it!" When he noses or paws the pot, click your clicker and lift the pot to reward him with the treat.

3. After your puppy catches on, which shouldn't take long, hold the pot in place and keep encouraging him until he paws at it. Tap his wrist or cue "**shake**" (page 60) to give him the idea to use his paw. Reward any paw contact by clicking and lifting the pot.

4. Add two more pots (mark the scented one so you don't forget which one it is!) In a soft voice, tell your puppy to "find it!"

5. Hold the pots in place while your puppy sniffs them so he doesn't knock them over in his exuberance. Use the pitch of your voice to calm your puppy as he diligently sniffs each pot, and to excite him when he shows interest in the correct one. If your puppy loses interest, quickly lift and set back down the correct pot to show him the treat.

6. If your puppy paws at an incorrect pot, do not lift it; instead say "whoops" and encourage him to keep looking.

7. When your puppy indicates the correct pot, click and lift the pot so he can get his reward!

WHAT TO EXPECT: Be encouraging with your puppy and avoid saying "no" when he indicates a wrong pot. Only practice a few times per session and end with a successful attempt, even if you have to go back to using just one pot to get that success.

TROUBLESHOOTING

MY PUPPY IS NOT INTERESTED IN SNIFFING THE FLOWER POT

Your puppy may not be smelling the scent of the treat. To make sure he smells the treat, take an aromatic treat (such as a piece of a hot dog) and use duct tape to fasten it to the inside of the pot, right up against the hole in the base.

TIP! Practice success, ignore the rest. Avoid telling your puppy "no" if he chooses incorrectly.

"Is it chowtime?
Did you call me?
Wait for me!"

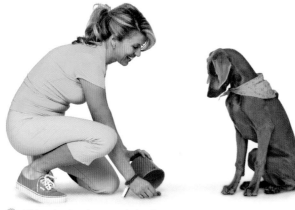

1 Hide a treat under a scented pot.

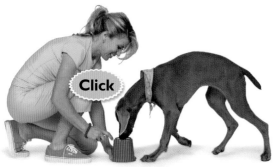 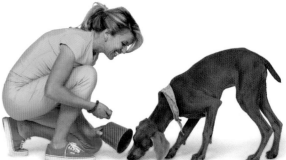

2 When your puppy noses the pot, click your clicker . . .   and lift the pot.

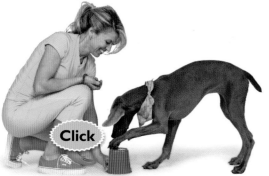 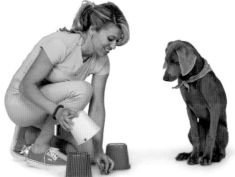

3 Hold the pot in place and don't click until your puppy paws it.

4 Add two more pots.

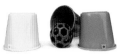

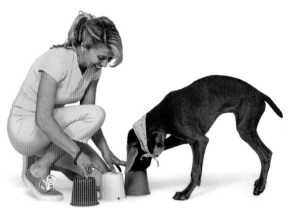

5 Hold the pots in place while your puppy sniffs each one.

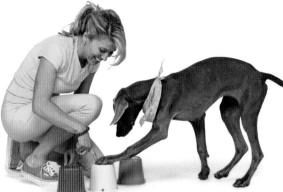

6 If your puppy indicates an incorrect pot, do not lift it. Encourage him to keep looking.

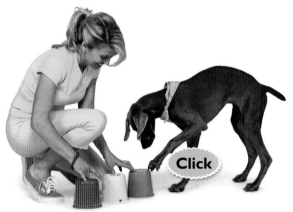

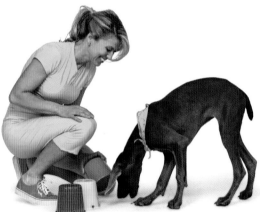

7 When your puppy indicates the correct pot, click . . .

and lift the pot so he can take the treat.

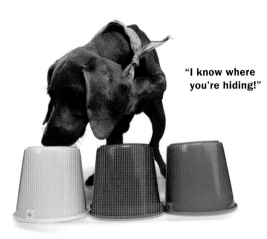

"I know where you're hiding!"

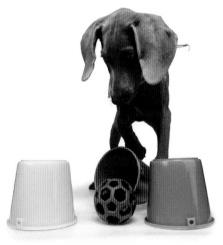

Find the Hidden Veggies

Hide veggies, treats, or kibble around your house, and teach your puppy to seek out as many as she can. This trick will teach your puppy to use her nose, and will keep her occupied for a few minutes!

"I'm really good at this trick. I know all the hiding places!"

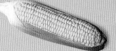

TEACH IT:

1 You could use treats or kibble for this trick, but fruits and vegetables as hidden treats offer a low-calorie alternative and are just as much fun. Hold a veggie to your puppy's nose and tell her "scent" to indicate the scent she is to search. Toss the veggie a short distance away on the floor and send her to "find it!" Praise her when she does.

2 Repeat this game again, making it a little harder. Place the veggie a little farther away or above the ground on a coffee table or stairs.

3 Place a few veggies around the room. If your puppy seems confused, encourage her by running with her toward a veggie. Increase the difficulty of hiding places as your puppy improves, but make sure she is still having good success, as you don't want her to become frustrated and give up.

WHAT TO EXPECT: This is a wonderful enrichment activity for puppies, as it teaches them to use their scenting and hunting abilities!

TROUBLESHOOTING

MY PUPPY GIVES UP TOO QUICKLY
The object is not to outwit your puppy, but to make her successful. Progress slowly so your puppy builds confidence in her ability. Over time, she will enjoy greater challenges. Strong-smelling treats will also be easier to find.

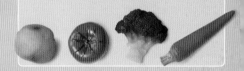

TIP! Some favorite raw veggies: carrots, green beans, corn, broccoli, potatoes, brussels sprouts, cauliflower, turnips, squash, sugar snap peas. Apples and bananas are favorite fruits!

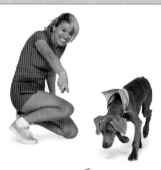

1 Toss a treat and have your puppy "find it!"

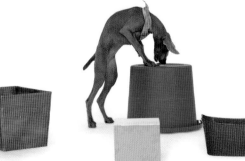

2 Hide the treat farther away or off the ground.

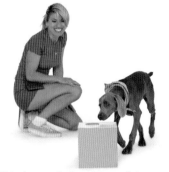

3 Hide several treats around the room.

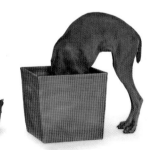

See how many your puppy can find!

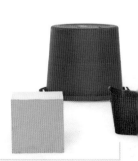

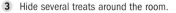

Close the Door

Close

Teach your puppy to push a door shut.
This skill also works to close a drawer,
cabinet, or toy box lid.

"I slam doors all the
time. I like to help."

TEACH IT:

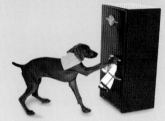

1. Before you start, you may wish to tape some cardboard on your door, as during the learning stage puppies will often scratch at the door. Open the door a few inches (cm) and hold a treat against the door at your puppy's nose height. Encourage him to "close, get it!" When he shows interest in the treat, raise the treat a little higher against the door, just out of his reach. In an attempt to get the treat your puppy will probably put his front paws up on the door to lift himself higher. This will result in his slamming the door closed. Click your clicker the instant he puts one or both paws against the door.

2. Let your puppy have the treat you were holding against the door. It is best to give him the treat while he still has his paws against the door rather than after he has dropped back to the floor.

3. Once your puppy has the hang of this, try merely tapping the door to get him to push on it. Click and reward him for pushing the door closed. Finally, send your puppy to "close" the door from a distance. Don't be surprised if he slams it shut in his eagerness!

WHAT TO EXPECT: Most puppies will enjoy slamming a door shut, and can learn this trick in a week.

TROUBLESHOOTING

MY PUPPY WAS FRIGHTENED BY THE BANG OF THE SLAMMING DOOR
Use this as a learning experience to accustom your puppy to loud sounds. This is an important part of socializing your puppy.

TIP! Use this same skill to teach your puppy to close a drawer or kitchen cabinet.

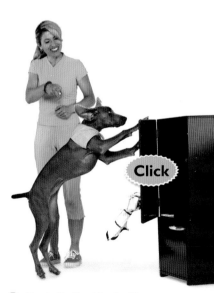

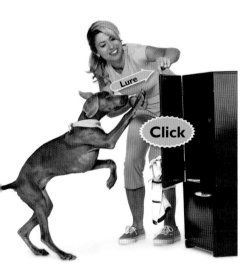

1. Hold a treat against the door and raise it just out of your puppy's reach. Click when he puts his paws on the door.

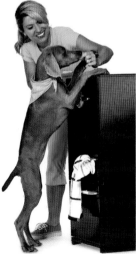

2. Give him a treat while he is in the correct position.

3. Now try it without the food lure.

Turn On a Tap Light

Teach your puppy to press a tap light on the floor to turn it on. We use a generic cue of "target" for this trick, as we can later adapt this skill for other applications.

**"Light on. Light off.
Light on. Light off.
Light on. Light off."**

1. Place a large tap light on the floor. During the learning phase it is helpful to tape it down so it doesn't move.

2. Let your puppy know that you have treats in your treat bag so that you have his interest. Hold your clicker ready in your hand, and tap the light to get your puppy's attention on it.

3. Your puppy will probably sniff the button and touch it with his nose. You don't want to reward the nose sniff, because the behavior we are trying to teach is a paw touch. But you do want to encourage your puppy to continue to interact with the tap light. So when he sniffs it, encourage him by saying "good! get it! keep going!" and tap the light again.

4. Out of frustration, your puppy will probably eventually scratch at the light. Be ready with your clicker and click the instant his paw even barely touches the light.

5. Immediately give a treat to your puppy. Optimally, you want to give the treat while he is in the correct position—with his paw on the light.

6. If your puppy never scratches at the light, there is another method you can try. Use a food treat to lure him forward and try to get him to accidentally step on the light, or even just barely touch it with his paw.

7. The instant he touches the light with his paw, click your clicker and also release the treat in your hand—at the same time.

8. Once your puppy starts to understand this trick, stand up and move a little away from the light, and send him to turn it on with the cue word "target!"

WHAT TO EXPECT: This is a fun trick for puppies once they get the hang of it. If you are very accurate with the timing of your clicker, your puppy can get the hang of this trick in a few days.

TROUBLESHOOTING

I CAN'T LURE MY PUPPY TO ACCIDENTALLY STEP ON THE LIGHT
Try this: Instead of affixing the light to the floor, affix it instead to a small wooden crate. Then lure your puppy to put his front paws onto the box. He will have a smaller space to put his paws, and will therefore be more likely to accidentally step on the light.

MY PUPPY IS NOT PRESSING THE LIGHT HARD ENOUGH TO TURN IT ON
In the beginning, reward him just for touching the light with his paw. Once he understands this well, withhold the treat and keep telling him "target!" He will probably become frustrated and hit the light harder—reward that!

TIP! During the learning phase, remove the batteries from the tap light, as the light can be an inadvertent reward marker signal to your puppy. It is better for you to control the reward marker with a clicker.

"Once I stepped on a bug but then he stopped moving."

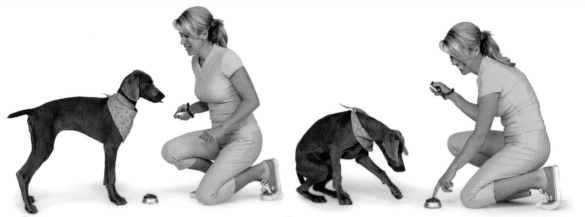

1 Affix a large tap light to the floor.

2 Touch it to get your puppy's interest.

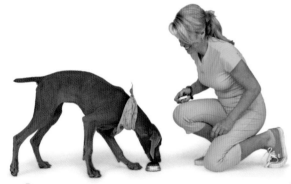

3 Don't reward a nose touch, but do encourage your puppy to keep interacting with the light.

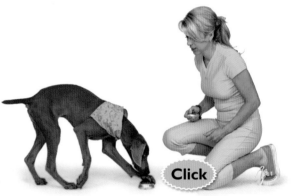

4 Your puppy will eventually scratch at the light. Click that!

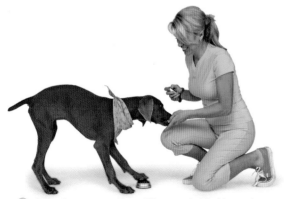

5 Reward your puppy. If possible, reward while his paw is on the light.

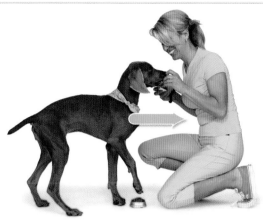

6 Lure your puppy to accidentally step on the light.

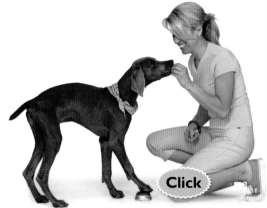

7 Click and release the treat at the same time.

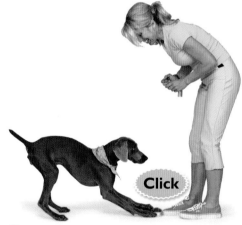

8 Stand up and cue your puppy with "target."

"I throwed up."

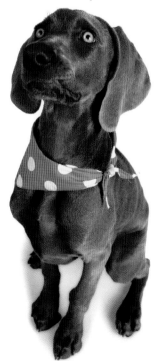

Chapter 5

Shape Behavior

"Can I eat them now?"

Clickers can mark a behavior very precisely, and are therefore used hand-in-hand with a training technique called **shaping**. With shaping, we break a behavior into baby steps, and we start by rewarding the most basic component of the trick. Once the puppy is repeatedly successful, we up the ante and only reward an attempt that comes closer to the goal.

Shaping is an especially effective technique to use with puppies. Puppies have short attention spans and a hard time focusing. They move very quickly, and become frustrated or distracted quicker than adult dogs. Shaping allows you to reward your puppy for just the smallest baby step toward the goal behavior. In this way, your puppy experiences a lot of successes—and a lot of treats—which maintain her focus and motivation to keep trying.

In using shaping to teach a puppy to fetch, for example, the first baby step could be to have the puppy merely touch a ball by your feet. Reward that simple behavior over and over (marking it precisely with a clicker each time). Once your puppy gets the hang of this, then require a little more of her; ask her to pick up the ball. Gradually place the ball farther away, until your puppy learns to fetch it from across the room!

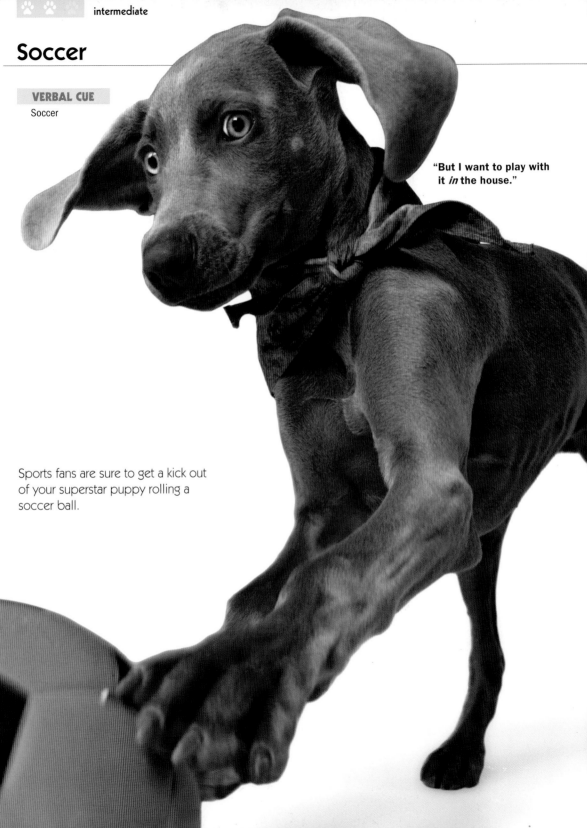

Soccer

VERBAL CUE

Soccer

"But I want to play with it *in* the house."

Sports fans are sure to get a kick out of your superstar puppy rolling a soccer ball.

1. Familiarize yourself with the shaping method of training (page 128). Have your clicker ready in your hand, and some treats in your treat bag. Place a soccer ball in an empty room. Your puppy will probably come over to investigate this new object, but if not, roll it a little and encourage her by saying "soccer! Get it!"

2. The instant your puppy touches the ball, click your clicker and follow up immediately with a treat.

3. If your puppy does not touch the ball, show her a treat and place it under the ball. When your puppy reaches for the treat, she will inadvertently touch the ball—click that! There is no need to give her a treat from your pocket, as she should have gotten the treat under the ball at the same time you clicked.

4. Once your puppy understands to touch the soccer ball, it is time to up the ante and ask more from her. Wait for your puppy to interact with the ball for a few seconds before you click and treat. This is where your shaping skills will really come into play. Your puppy will probably touch the ball once, and look at you, expecting a click. When she doesn't hear the click, she'll try again and push the ball harder with her nose, or push it with her paw—click either of those actions and follow with a treat. If your puppy gets frustrated, go back to rewarding her for just touching the ball.

WHAT TO EXPECT: Teaching the soccer trick is a great way for both you and your puppy to learn the art of shaping. Practice daily and in a week your puppy can be on her way to the World Cup!

TROUBLESHOOTING

MY PUPPY BITES THE BALL

During the learning phase you want to avoid saying "no" to your puppy, as that could discourage her from trying new things. Never click when your puppy is biting; wait for her to move the ball without biting. You could also try using a large, hard plastic ball, which your puppy will be unable to bite. You can find these balls as part of a toy bowling set.

TIP! When your puppy is successful 75 percent of the time, up the ante and require more of her.

"No! I won't, I won't, I won't!

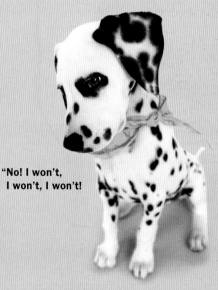

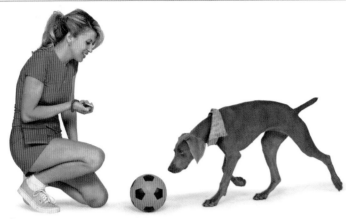

1 Your puppy will want to investigate this new object.

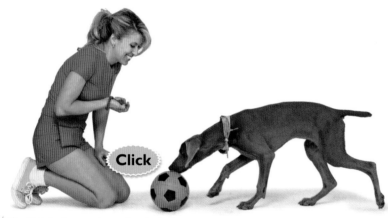

2 Click the instant she touches the ball.

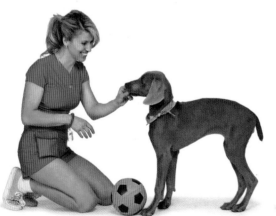

Follow up with a treat.

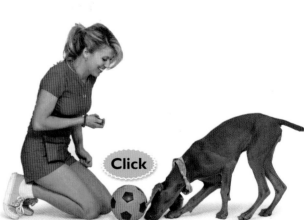

3 Place a treat under the ball. Click when your puppy touches the ball while reaching for the treat.

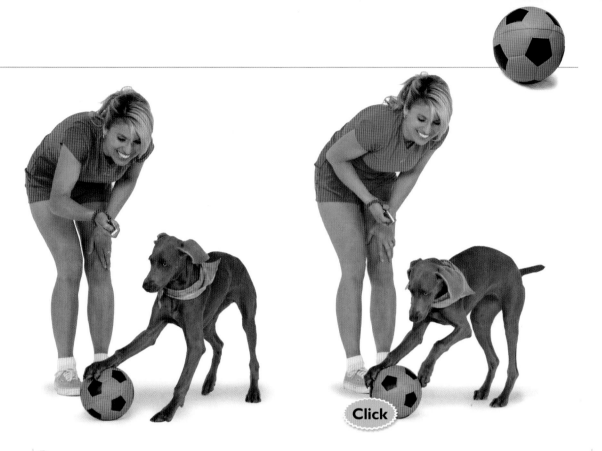

4 Have your puppy interact with the ball for longer periods of time before you reward her.

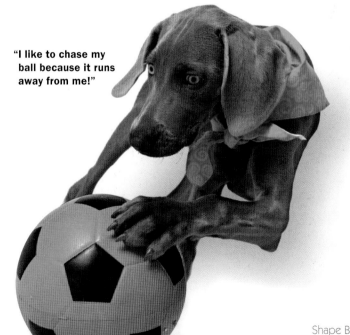

"I like to chase my ball because it runs away from me!"

Beginning Fetch

"I find all *kinds* of stuff to bring to my owner."

Teach your puppy to fetch an object. This important trick is not only useful, but it conditions your puppy to work for you.

NATURAL RETRIEVERS

1 Puppies have natural retrieving instincts, so we can take advantage of this inclination. Start with a high-value toy (a favorite toy) that your puppy enjoys putting in his mouth.

2 Get your puppy interested in the toy by playing with it. Then toss the toy a short distance away and say "fetch!"

3 Once your puppy picks up the toy, encourage him to bring it back to you by patting your legs, calling to him, acting excited, or backing away from him.

4 When he brings the toy to you, take the toy, give him a treat, and then give the toy right back to him. It is important that your puppy knows he will not lose his toy by bringing it to you, or he may become reluctant to bring it to you!

RELUCTANT RETRIEVERS

5 With very young puppies, or dog breeds that have not been bred as retrievers, you may not be successful with the first method of teaching fetch. In this case we can use the more incremental method of shaping (page 128). Be ready with your clicker in your hand. Play with your puppy's favorite plush toy, moving it around, and tossing it in the air. The instant your puppy puts his mouth on the toy, click your clicker, and quickly follow up with a treat.

6 Once your puppy is successful biting the toy, up the ante and require more of your puppy to get the click. Toss the toy playfully on the ground, and click him for biting it. The next time, up the ante again and don't click until he picks up the toy and turns his head toward you. As always, each click is followed by a treat.

7 Once your puppy is successful at the short fetch, toss the toy farther and say "fetch!". Click your clicker when your puppy returns with the toy and give him a treat.

WHAT TO EXPECT: Most puppies enjoy carrying things in their mouths, and will understand the basics of fetch within a week. Puppies are easily distracted, so don't increase distance too quickly.

TROUBLESHOOTING

MY PUPPY GETS THE TOY AND RUNS OFF WITH IT
Never chase your puppy when he is playing keep-away. Lure him back with a treat, or run away from him to encourage him to chase you. Have a second toy to get his attention.

I CAN'T GET MY PUPPY TO EVEN PICK UP THE TOY
Start by clicking and rewarding your puppy for just touching or sniffing the toy. If he doesn't even do that, start by clicking him for putting his head down toward the toy. Start small, and up the ante as your puppy gets the hang of each step.

TIP! If at any point your puppy is repeatedly unsuccessful, return to the previous step.

"Yay! A car ride! Yay-yay-yay-yay!"

NATURAL RETRIEVERS

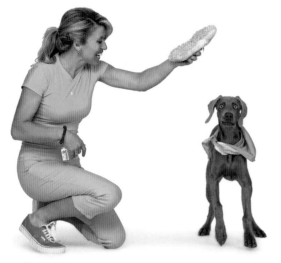

1 Play with a toy your puppy likes.

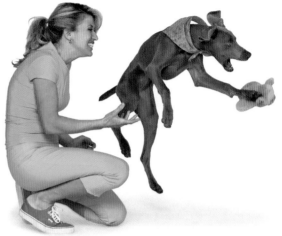

2 Once he seems interested in the toy, toss it playfully.

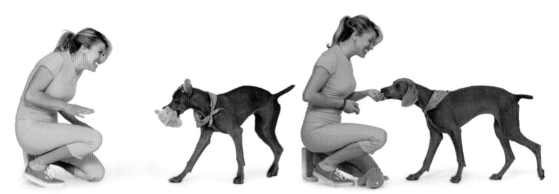

3 Encourage your puppy to bring it back to you.

4 Give him a treat, and also let him have his toy again.

RELUCTANT RETRIEVERS

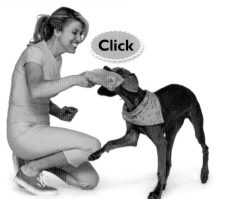

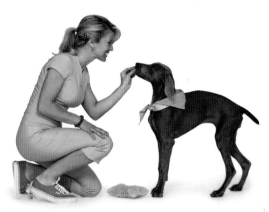

5 The instant your puppy puts his mouth on the toy, click . . .   and follow up with a treat.

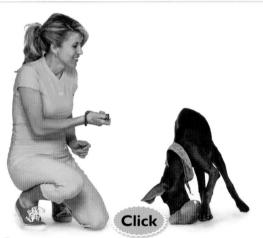

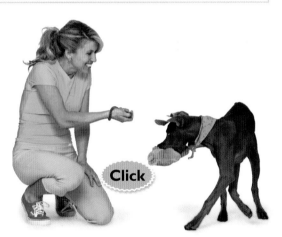

6 Up the ante and toss the toy on the ground. Click your puppy for biting it.

Up the ante again and wait for him to pick up the toy and turn toward you. Click that.

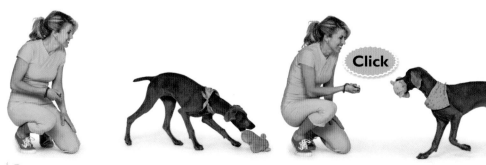

7 Toss the toy farther away.   Click when your puppy returns with the toy.

Fetch the Newspaper to Hand

VERBAL CUE

Fetch

Once your puppy has learned beginning fetch, increase the difficulty by teaching her to deliver the item into your hand. Teach her to fetch the daily newspaper.

"This is an important job and I have to do it every day."

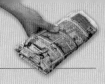

1 First, teach your puppy **beginning fetch** (page 134). Train indoors to start, as there will be fewer distractions for your puppy. Secure a section of the newspaper with a rubber band and toss it playfully for your puppy. Tell her to "fetch! Get the paper!" Once she picks up the paper, pat your legs to encourage her to come back to you.

2 Once your puppy is consistently fetching the newspaper, you can begin to teach her to deliver the paper directly into your hand. In order to teach her this, you have to arrange for her to be successful, and then reward her for that success. You have to create a situation where she actually delivers the newspaper into your hand, without dropping it. This is going to take some quick action on your part. As your puppy returns to you with the newspaper, keep your left foot planted and take a big step backward with your right foot. This will draw your puppy in closer to you.

3 When your puppy is close enough, keep your left foot planted and lunge forward with your right foot. Try to catch the newspaper before it hits the floor.

4 If you manage to catch the newspaper, praise your puppy profusely, and give her a big treat!

5 If you aren't able to catch the newspaper before it falls to the floor, you'll want to try to get your puppy to pick it up again. You are teaching your puppy that her job is not done yet. Hold a treat in your hand to motivate your puppy, and point to the newspaper and encourage her to "fetch!" If she doesn't get the hint, wiggle the newspaper a bit to get her interest.

6 Only reward your puppy if you take the newspaper from her mouth. If you absolutely can't get your puppy to pick up the newspaper again, then walk away without picking up the newspaper, and try again later.

WHAT TO EXPECT: Puppies have a habit of dropping items after they lose interest. Be consistent in teaching your puppy to fetch the newspaper all the way to your hand. Once a puppy has learned to fetch, she can learn to fetch to hand in another week. Teach your puppy to fetch the daily newspaper to your hand by first standing in your driveway, very close to the newspaper, and having her bring it to you. Gradually stand closer and closer to your front door, increasing the distance of the fetch.

TROUBLESHOOTING

MY PUPPY SHREDS THE NEWSPAPER!
You'll want to nip this in the bud. Toys are for chewing on, but the newspaper belongs to you, and is not a toy. During the learning phase, wrap the folded newspaper in packing tape, so your puppy builds a habit of fetching it, rather than destroying it.

TIP! In dog training vernacular "cookie" means a food treat. "Do you want a cookie?"

"I have a pink collar and I like it. Sometimes I don't want to wear it though."

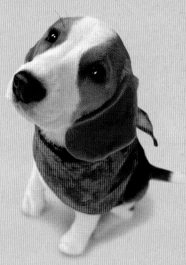

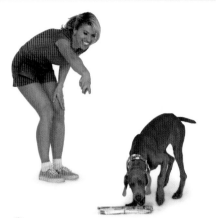
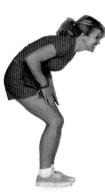
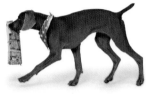

1 Secure the newspaper with a rubber band. Toss it playfully and tell your puppy to "fetch! Get the paper!"

Pat your legs and encourage her back to you.

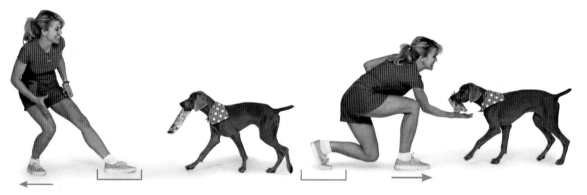

2 Keep your left foot planted; step back with your right foot.

3 Keep your left foot planted; lunge forward with your right foot and catch the newspaper.

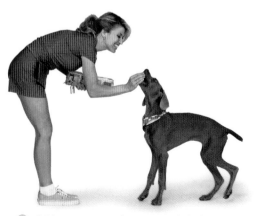

4 Celebrate your puppy's success and give her a big treat!

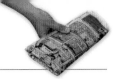

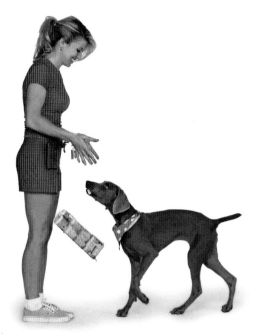

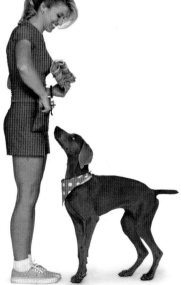

5 If the paper falls to the floor . . .

try to get your puppy to pick it up from the floor.

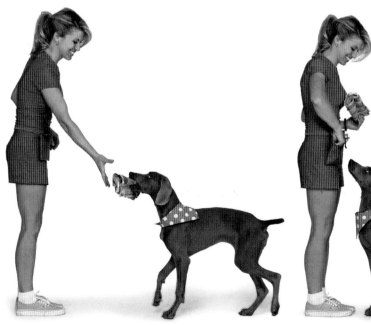

6 Take the paper from your puppy's mouth.

Reward your puppy only if you take the newspaper from her mouth.

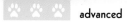

Open the Door

VERBAL CUE
Open

Tie a rope or dish towel to the door handle, and teach your puppy to pull it open!

"This is where we keep the dog biscuits!"

TEACH IT:

1 Familiarize yourself with the shaping method of training (page 128). Tie a treat inside a dish towel to entice your puppy, and wiggle it on the floor. When your puppy puts his mouth on the towel, click your clicker and then give him a treat.

2 Next, try to get your puppy to hold on to the towel for a second. Once he has bitten the towel, continue to wiggle it and pull it a little to engage his prey drive. Whenever he holds on to the towel for two seconds, click and give him a treat.

3 Tie the dish towel on the door handle. It might help to again tie a treat inside the towel. Wiggle the towel and click your puppy for any interaction with the towel, even if it is only touching the towel with his nose while sniffing for the treat.

4 Up the ante and wait for your puppy to bite the towel before clicking and treating.

5 Once your puppy is successfully biting the towel, hold off on clicking until he pulls the towel a little. Don't ask for much; click just the slightest tug at first.

6 As your puppy shows consistent success with each step, you can ask a little more of him. In its final stage, upon your "open" cue your puppy should pull hard enough on the towel to open the door.

WHAT TO EXPECT: This trick is a little more difficult to teach than it may at first appear. Your skill as a trainer will be challenged as you work through the process of teaching this trick. The most important thing to remember is that you want your puppy to have as many successes (clicks) as possible, so raise your criteria for success in very slow and small increments. You will probably want your puppy to have ten to thirty successes on each step before you progress to the next step.

TROUBLESHOOTING

MY PUPPY STALLED OUT ON A STEP
It's not uncommon for a puppy to stall out. Often they will get stuck nosing the towel but not biting it, or will get stuck biting it but not pulling. In those cases, click your puppy for doing the current step twice in a row. So, for example, if he bites the towel, don't click that but instead wait for him to bite it a second time and click that. Be observant though, and click if his first attempt is actually a pull.

TIP! This trick can also be used to open drawers, cabinets, mailboxes, and toy box lids.

"I like to open doors myself so my owner doesn't have to help me."

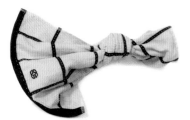

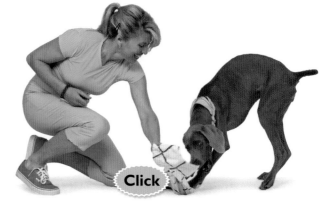

1 Tie a treat inside a dish towel.

Wiggle the dish towel to get your puppy's interest. Click when your puppy bites it, and give him a treat.

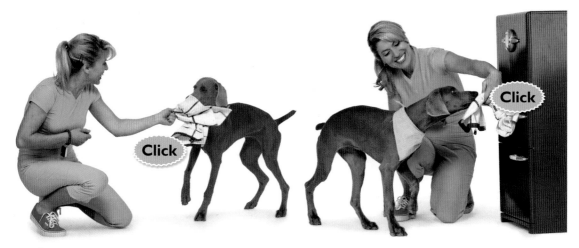

2 Tug on the towel a little to get your puppy to hold on to it longer. After two seconds of holding, click and treat.

3 Click your puppy for sniffing the treat tied inside the dish towel.

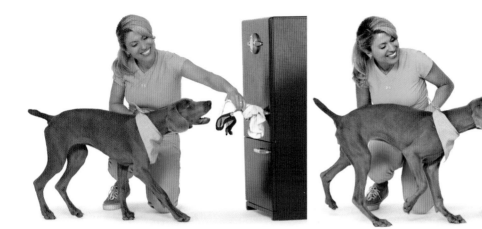

4 Up the ante and . . .

wait until your puppy bites the towel before clicking.
Follow each click with a treat.

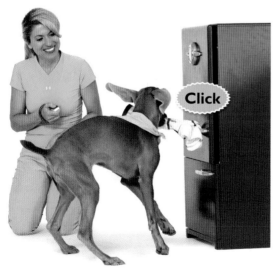

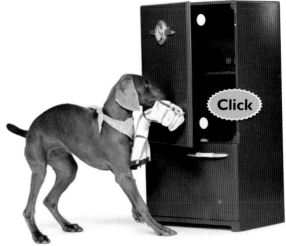

5 Now see if your puppy can do a slight tug.

6 Eventually your puppy will be able to pull hard enough to
open the door.

Hide Your Eyes

"I'm not peeking!"

In this adorable trick, your puppy hides his eyes by hooking his paw over his muzzle.

1. During the learning phase your puppy will only touch his muzzle with his paw for a quick instant. Your success in teaching this this trick will rely heavily on your precise timing with your clicker. Take a piece of tape and stick it on your puppy's head or muzzle. Cellophane tape doesn't generally have enough adhesive to stick to your puppy for long, so you may want to try a more adhesive tape. If your puppy has long fur, stick the tape on your pants a few times to lessen its adhesion.

2. Encourage your puppy to "cover, get it!" The tape will be annoying to him, and he will naturally swipe at his face with his paw. Be ready with your clicker and click the instant his paw touches his face.

3. Follow up your click very quickly with a treat. If the swipe at his head did not dislodge the tape, then your puppy will continue to be distracted by it. He therefore may not even realize that you are offering him a treat. So as soon as you click, put that treat right into his mouth. Keep sessions short, and only do five to ten repetitions of it at a time. Once your puppy has done about 100 total repetitions, go on to the next step.

4. After doing several repetitions in a row with the tape, try one without the tape. Just tap the spot on your puppy's head where you normally stick the tape, and again say "cover!"

5. If your puppy actually does swipe at his face, then click and treat. If not, regress to using the tape again. It is often the case that the trainer will have to go back and forth many times between tapping the puppy's head, and then regressing to using the tape again.

6. Eventually you will not need to use the tape or even tap your puppy's head. Simply giving the verbal cue and hand signal will be enough to get him to cover his eyes with his paw.

WHAT TO EXPECT: This method of training is so natural that your puppy should be swiping the tape right away. After about a month, or 200 repetitions, your puppy should have the hang of an eye cover with the aid of the tape. It could take a lot longer, however, until he has it mastered without that aid.

TROUBLESHOOTING

MY PUPPY SHAKES HIS HEAD INSTEAD OF PAWING AT THE TAPE

Use a stronger adhesive tape so your puppy can't merely shake it off. Try sticking the tape in different places: above or below his eye or on top of his head.

MY PUPPY JUST SITS THERE WITH THE TAPE STUCK TO HIS NOSE!

Encourage your puppy to attack the tape, as he would a bug on his nose. Touch the tape to make him aware of it and use your voice to excite him, "Get it! Get it!"

TIP! Take your puppy on a trip or errand. It will be good for his social skills and he'll enjoy the change of scenery.

"This trick is hard 'cause sometimes I fall over."

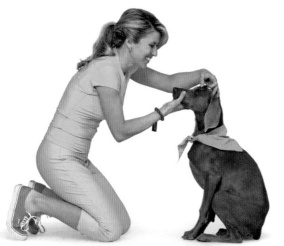

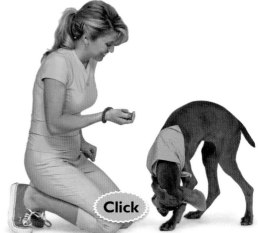

1 Stick a piece of tape to your puppy's head or muzzle.

2 Click the instant your puppy's paw touches his face.

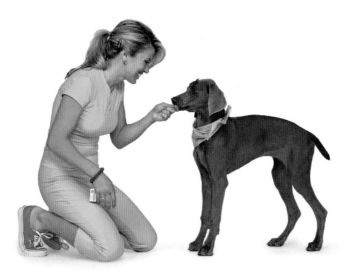

3 Follow the click by putting a treat in your puppy's mouth.

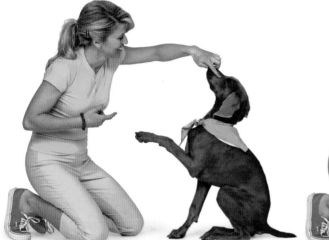

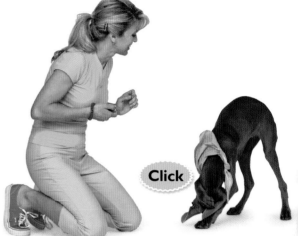

4 Tap the spot on your puppy's head where you normally stick the tape, and cue "cover!"

5 Often the trainer will have to alternate between tapping the puppy's head and using the tape.

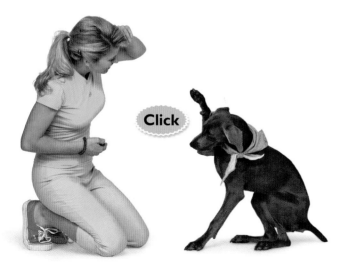

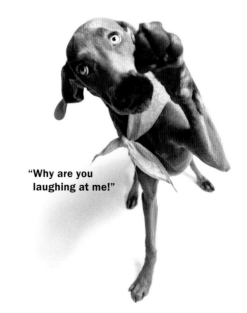

"Why are you laughing at me!"

6 Give the hand signal and tell you puppy to "cover!"

Skateboard

VERBAL CUE

Skateboard

Your puppy can learn to push a skateboard by placing three paws on the skateboard and pushing with her remaining back paw.

"I like to get on top of things."

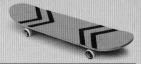

1. Familiarize yourself with the shaping method of training (page 128). Hold the skateboard in place with your foot, and lure your puppy to put her front **paws up** on top (page 48). The moment both of her paws are on the skateboard, click, and let her have the treat.

2. Now teach your puppy to put a third paw on the skateboard. Keep your foot on the skateboard to keep it from moving. Hold your clicker and a treat in one hand, and hold this hand near your puppy's nose to keep her head and front paws in place. Move your body to the side of the skateboard where your puppy has her back feet. Tap her rear leg which is closes to the skateboard to give her the idea to move her leg onto the skateboard. When she does, click and let her have the treat from your front hand.

3. Once your puppy understands the goal of having three paws on the skateboard, it's time to get it rolling. Attach a leash around the front wheels. Have your puppy put three paws on the skateboard, and keep her attention by holding a treat slightly ahead of her. Pull very slowly on the leash. The instant her fourth paw leaves the ground, click and give her a treat. Continue pulling, clicking, and treating. You should be clicking every couple of seconds, corresponding with every time her fourth paw leaves the ground. Remember to give a treat after every click.

4. Remove the leash and walk backward. Cue "skateboard" while coaxing your puppy to push the skateboard toward you.

WHAT TO EXPECT: Puppies can learn the objective of three paws on the skateboard in a matter of days. The coordination of pushing with their fourth paw may take an additional several weeks or even several months. Bulldogs and Parson Russell breeds seem to love this trick best!

TROUBLESHOOTING

MY PUPPY SOMETIMES STEPS ON THE END OF THE SKATEBOARD, MAKING IT FLIP UP

If this is scaring your puppy, you can attach foam blocks to the underside of either end of the skateboard, preventing it from flipping up. If your puppy is not scared, however, do not make an adjustment to the skateboard, but instead allow your puppy the time and experimentation to figure out on her own how to balance on the skateboard.

TIP! Teach skateboard on a smooth surface. Cracks in the concrete or irregularities in an asphalt parking lot will stall the skateboard.

"Do you know what meatballs are? They're really, really, really good!"

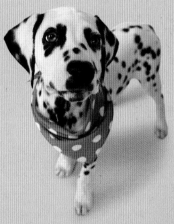

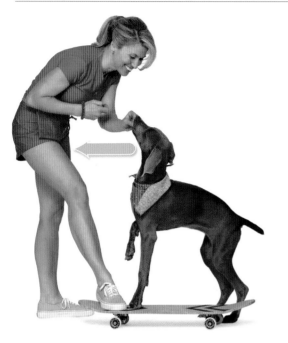

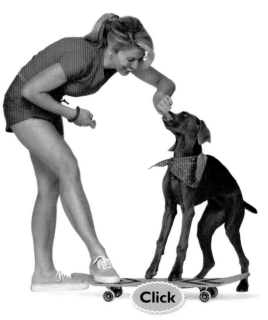

1 Hold the skateboard with your foot and lure your puppy to put her front paws on top.

The moment both of her paws come onto the skateboard, click and give her the treat.

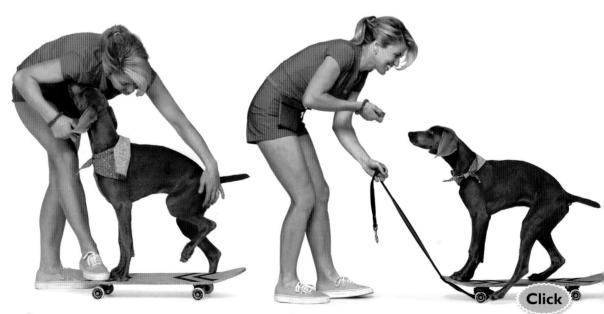

2 Keep a treat at nose height, and click when your puppy's third paw comes on the skateboard.

3 Attach a leash to the skateboard and reward your puppy for lifting her fourth paw.

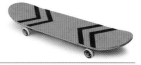

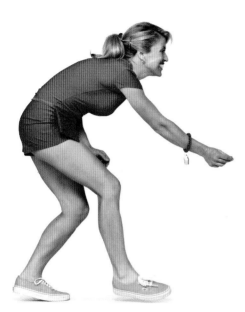

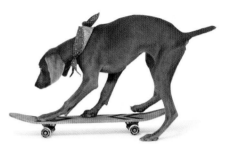

4 Remove the leash and coax your puppy toward you.

"Faster! Faster!"

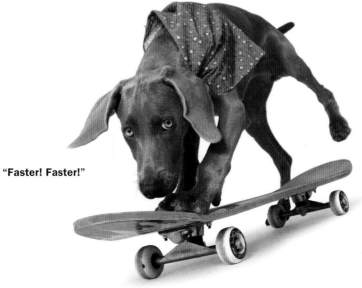

Chapter 6:

Chaining

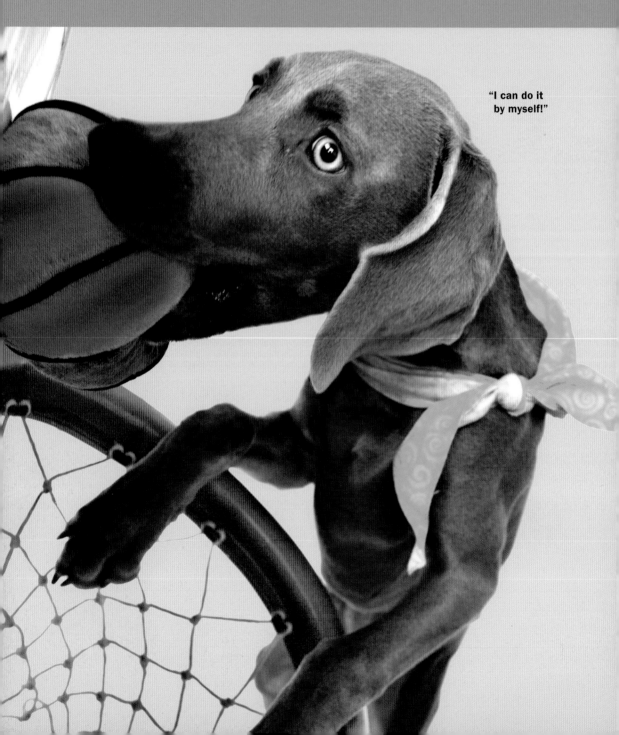

"I can do it
by myself!"

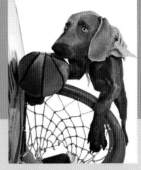

Link

Link several simple tricks together to produce one really impressive chained trick! When teaching a chained trick, first teach each component of the trick as separate behavior. Later, have your puppy perform the behaviors in sequence, and then give a name to the entire sequence.

Dunking a basketball into a net is an example of a chained trick. It combines three simple behaviors:

- **Fetch** the ball
- Put **paws up** on the rim
- **Drop** the ball through the net

Once the puppy is able to do each of the behaviors individually, then practice them in sequence. A new cue word, "dunk," is introduced to represent the entire chain, so that the puppy comes to think of the entire chain as one trick.

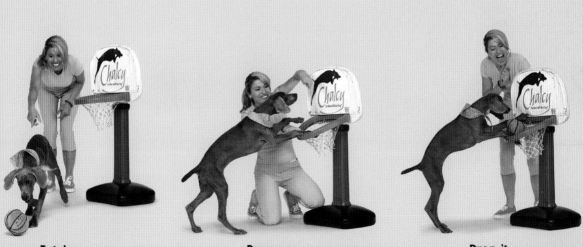

Fetch   **Paws up**   **Drop it**

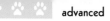

Tidy Up Toys into Toy Box

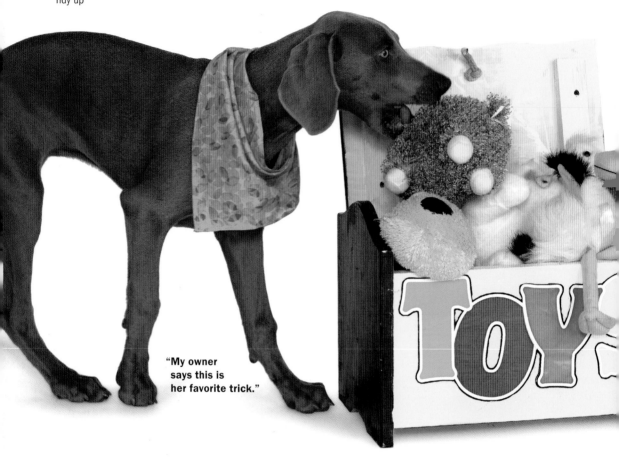

"My owner
says this is
her favorite trick."

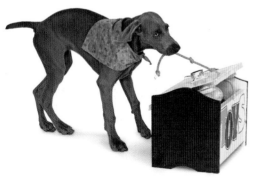

Your puppy opens his toy box lid, puts his
toys inside, and closes the lid. Add this trick
to your puppy's daily chores, and you'll be
the envy of the neighborhood!

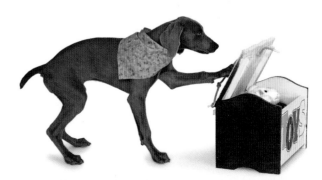

PUT AWAY THE TOY

1 Hold a treat in one hand, and your clicker in the other. Toss a plush toy and instruct your puppy to **fetch** (page 134).

2 When your puppy returns with the toy, hold the treat a few inches (cm) above the open toy box, near the edge farthest from your puppy. When he opens his mouth for the treat, the toy should fall right in. The instant this happens, click and let him have the treat!

3 In the beginning, if your puppy's toy drops near the toy box but not quite inside, let him have the treat but don't click your clicker. As he improves, only click and treat when the toy falls inside the toy box.

OPEN THE LID

4 Attach a thick, knotted rope to the toy box lid on the edge nearest the opening. Wedge a toy under the lid so that stays partially open. Set your puppy behind the toy box and wiggle the rope. When your puppy sniffs or bites or touches the rope, click and give him a treat. If your puppy is not interested in the rope, try rubbing some hot dog scent on it.

5 After your puppy understands that he needs to touch the rope to get a click, ask a little more of him. This time, don't click when he touches the rope. He will probably touch it a second time. Then he may become frustrated and bite the rope—click that!

6 Next, try to get your puppy to pull slightly on to the rope. Encourage him by saying "open! Get it! Get it!" Click and treat him for the slightest pull.

7 Finally, remove the toy wedged under the lid so your puppy can pull the lid open all by himself!

CLOSE THE LID

8 We don't use a clicker for this one, as both of your hands will be occupied, and the bang of the closing lid will serve as the success indicator. Kneel down and hold the lid partially open with one hand and use a treat in your other hand to lure your puppy to step on the lid. Tell your puppy "close."

9 When he steps on the lid, allow it to fall closed and let him take the treat from your hand. He should still have his front paws on the lid when he receives his reward. If the bang of the lid startles him, you can lay a dish towel across the rim of the toy box to muffle the slam.

10 Gradually start with the lid farther and farther open, until your puppy figures out that the behavior you want is merely slamming the lid, and not necessarily stepping on it.

WHAT TO EXPECT: If your puppy already knows how to fetch, he can learn to drop the toy into the toy box within two or three weeks. Many puppies can learn to close the lid in a week, but opening the lid often takes longer to learn.

TROUBLESHOOTING

MY PUPPY IS SOMETIMES CONFUSED AND TAKES TOYS OUT OF THE BOX!
Your puppy is eager to please! "Whoops!" will alert your puppy that a mistake has been made.

MY PUPPY WANTS TO PLAY WITH THE TOY, AND NOT DROP IT
Use less desirable toys.

PUT IT ALL TOGETHER! Familiarize yourself with the process of chaining behaviors (page 154). First teach each of the components, and then teach the chain by first cueing "tidy up" and then cueing each of the components: "open," "fetch," "close."

PUT AWAY THE TOY

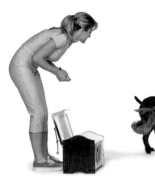 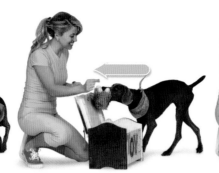 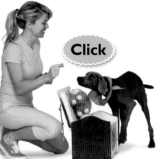

1 Toss a plush toy and have your puppy fetch.

2 Hold a treat above the back edge of the toy box.

Click the moment your puppy opens his mouth.

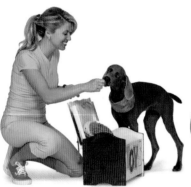 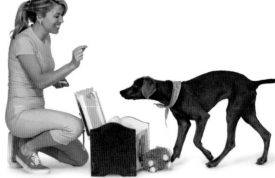

Let your puppy have the treat.

3 In the beginning, reward if the toy drops near the toy box.

OPEN THE LID

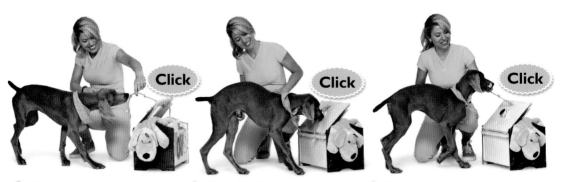

4 Click your puppy for sniffing or touching the rope.

5 Now wait until your puppy bites the rope before you click.

6 Then challenge your puppy to pull on the rope. Click and treat.

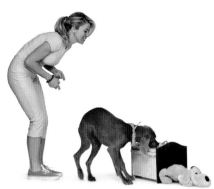

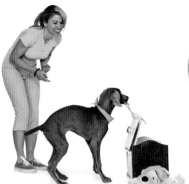

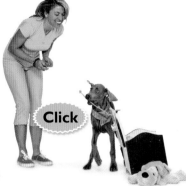

7 Remove the toy wedged under the lid.

Have your puppy open it all by himself!

Click and reward your puppy for pulling it open.

CLOSE THE LID

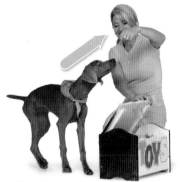

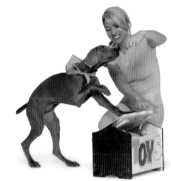

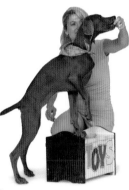

8 Hold the lid partially open and lure your puppy up.

This should cause him to step on the lid.

9 Reward him while his paws are on the lid.

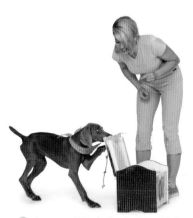

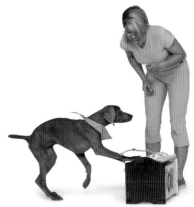

10 Increase difficulty by starting with the lid fully open.

Have your puppy slam it shut.

Litter in the Step Can

This one will really impress your friends! Teach your puppy to open the step can using the foot pedal, and watch her throw the trash inside.

"I check the trash can all the time to see if there is anything good in there"

DROP THE TRASH IN THE CAN

1 Hold a treat in one hand and your clicker in the other. Toss a plush toy and instruct your puppy to **fetch** (page 134).

2 When your puppy returns with the toy, use your clicker hand to hold open the step can lid. With your other hand, hold your treat against the step can lid. When she opens her mouth for the treat, the toy should fall right in the can. The instant she drops the toy, click and let her have the treat! In the beginning, if your puppy's toy drops near the step can, but not quite inside, let her have the treat but don't click your clicker. As she improves, you can challenge her by requiring the toy to make it inside the step can. You can help her by using your finger to gently coax the toy into the step can.

STEP ON THE FOOT PEDAL

3 If your puppy already knows how to **turn on a tap light** (page 124) you can temporarily affix the tap light onto the foot pedal to give her the idea to step on it. Otherwise, use a treat to lure your puppy forward so that she accidentally steps on the pedal. It can help to modify the foot pedal to make it larger.

4 Whenever your puppy accidently steps on the foot pedal, or even touches it, click and give her a treat. If possible, try to keep your treat steady so she remains on the foot pedal as she eats the treat.

5 As she improves, your puppy will learn to deliberately step on the foot pedal, and you should no longer need to lure her with a treat. Tell her "target" and when she steps on the pedal, click and treat.

WHAT TO EXPECT: This trick is actually not as hard to teach as you might think. Puppies seem to enjoy stepping on the foot pedal, and catch on to the concept in a few days. If you work at this trick several times a week, it will likely take a month before your puppy can do this on her own.

PUT IT ALL TOGETHER! Familiarize yourself with the process of chaining behaviors (page 154). Teach each component separately, and then teach your puppy to chain them together.

1 Hold the lid half way open, toss a toy, and cue your puppy "trash." She will probably slide the toy under the lid, and into the can. Click and reward that.

2 Then hold the lid slightly more closed and cue your puppy to fetch another toy. Your puppy may have some trouble this time, and may drop the toy on top of the lid. Once she has dropped the toy in the vicinity of the step can, cue her to step on the foot pedal with "target." When she does step on the foot pedal and open the lid, hold the lid open and cue her again to fetch the toy and drop it in the can. Click and treat only once the toy made it into the can.

3 You want your puppy to be successful as many times as possible, so this often means cheating a little to help your puppy. If your puppy holds the toy near the trash can, go ahead and use your finger to help it in. Then click and reward. If your puppy steps on the foot pedal, but then steps off of it, go ahead and hold the lid open a little so that she can get her toy in.

TROUBLESHOOTING

WHAT TYPE OF STEP CAN SHOULD I USE?
Use a step can with a flat lid, with no lip on it (as in the photo) so your puppy can use her nose to open it. A step can with a slow-closing lid will be helpful during the learning process.

DROP THE TRASH IN THE CAN

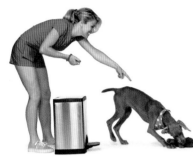 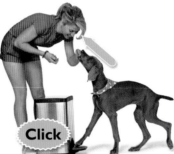 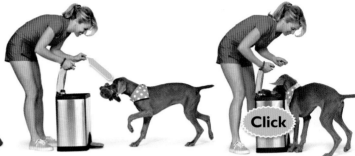

1 Have your puppy fetch a plush toy.

2 Hold the lid open with your clicker hand. Hold a treat near the lid.

Click when she opens her mouth.

STEP ON THE FOOT PEDAL

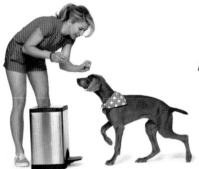 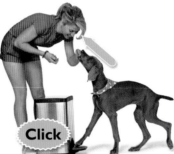 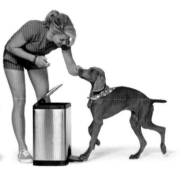

3 Lure your puppy near the foot pedal with a treat.

4 When your puppy accidentally touches the pedal, click.

Follow each click with a treat.

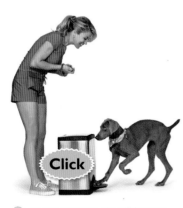 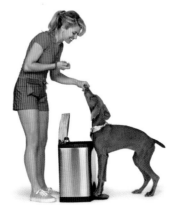

5 As she improves, she will learn to deliberately step on the pedal.

Reward while she has her paw on the pedal.

PUT IT ALL TOGETHER

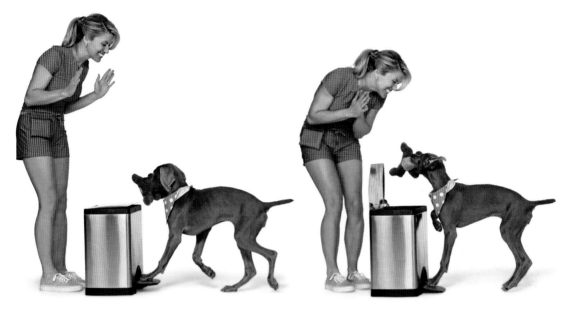

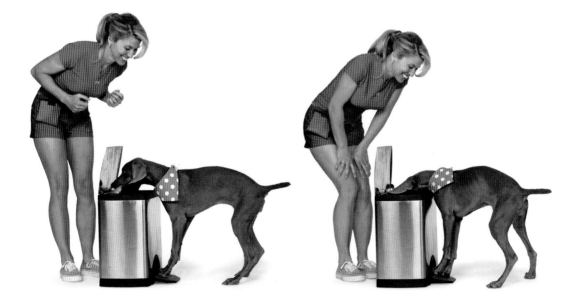

Soda from the Fridge

VERBAL CUE

Soda

"My owner says when I'm good for a whole day she'll give me a hamburger. I haven't gotten any hamburgers yet."

In this useful trick, your puppy opens the refrigerator door, fetches a soda, and returns to close the door.

GET THE SODA

1 Before you begin teaching this step, teach your puppy to **fetch** (page 134) and **fetch to hand** (page 138). Select a small, empty soda bottle that will be easy for your puppy to hold in his mouth. A foam can insulator may help him get a better grip on the bottle. Toss the bottle on the floor a few times for your puppy to fetch, to get him accustomed to carrying it.

2 Place the soda bottle on a low shelf in an open, uncluttered refrigerator and have your puppy fetch it from there.

OPEN THE REFRIGERATOR

3 Before you begin teaching this step, teach your puppy to **open a door** (page 142). Tie a dish towel to your refrigerator handle. Open the fridge door slightly as your puppy may not be strong enough and heavy enough to pull open the fridge's seal. Have your puppy pull the dish towel by cueing "open." Reward him for this step.

CLOSE THE REFRIGERATOR

4 Before you begin teaching this step, teach your puppy to **close a door** (page 122). Start with the refrigerator door only slightly open. Tap on the door at a height above your puppy's head, and cue him to "close." Reward him for this step.

WHAT TO EXPECT: Once your puppy is comfortable with all three steps, start to phase out the individual commands and use "soda" to represent the entire series. Now that your puppy knows the secret of the refrigerator, however, you may have to install a padlock!

PUT IT ALL TOGETHER! Familiarize yourself with the process of chaining behaviors (page 154). First teach each of the trick components, and then teach the chain by first cueing "soda" and then cueing each of the components: "open," "fetch," "close."

TROUBLESHOOTING

MY FLOOR IS GETTING SCRATCHED UP! Lightweight puppies and tile floors are a slippery combination as your puppy pulls the dish towel. Improve his traction with a doormat, or use a longer rope on the door handle to increase his angle of leverage.

"Here's what's fun: running with toilet paper"

GET THE SODA

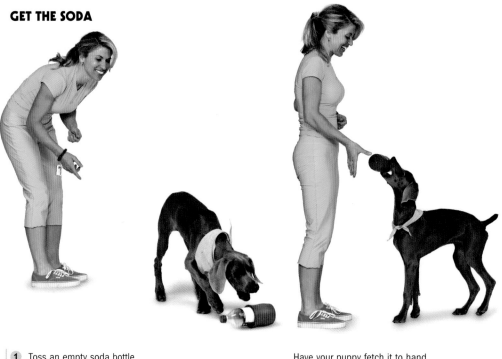

1 Toss an empty soda bottle.

Have your puppy fetch it to hand.

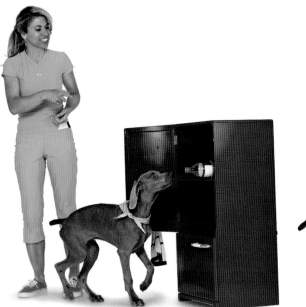
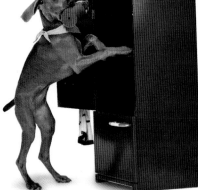

2 Place the bottle in the open refrigerator.

Have your puppy fetch it from there.

OPEN THE REFRIGERATOR

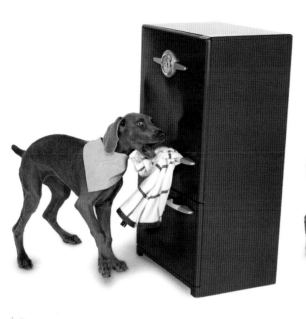

3 Tie a dish towel to the refrigerator handle.

Cue your puppy to "open."

CLOSE THE REFRIGERATOR

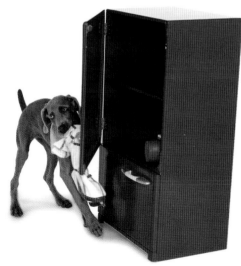

He will use the dish towel to open the door.

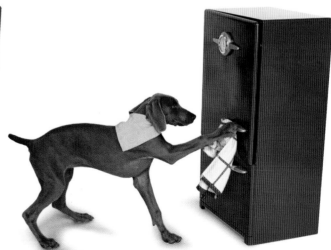

4 Tap the door and cue "close."

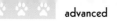

Mail from the Mailbox

VERBAL CUE

Get the mail

Teach your puppy
to open the
mailbox door,
retrieve the mail,
and close the door.

**"Here's what's
fun: ripping up
pieces of paper."**

GET THE MAIL

① Before teaching this trick, teach your puppy to **fetch** (page 134) and **fetch to hand** (page 138). Toss a rolled up piece of mail or newspaper on the floor, and have your puppy to fetch it a few times.

② Place the newspaper inside your open mailbox and tap it to direct your puppy's interest. Have him "fetch" and reward him when he brings it to you.

OPEN THE MAILBOX

③ Attach a knotted rope to the top of your mailbox door. Wiggle the rope. When your puppy sniffs or bites or touches the rope at all, click your clicker and give him a treat. If your puppy is not interested in the rope, try rubbing some hot dog scent on it.

④ Once your puppy understands that touching the rope earns him a click and a treat, make it a little harder. This time, don't click when he touches the rope. He will probably touch it a second time. Then he may become frustrated and bite the rope—click that!

⑤ Next, try to get your puppy to pull on to the rope. Encourage him by saying "open! Get it! Get it!" Click and treat him for the slightest pull.

⑥ Finally, try to get your puppy to pull the mailbox door all the way open before you click.

CLOSE THE MAILBOX

⑦ Remove the rope attached to the mailbox door, so as not to confuse your puppy. Tie together two large rubber bands and use them to hold the mailbox door a few inches (cm) open. The elasticity in the rubber bands will hold the door slightly open, but will not cause the mailbox to tip forward if your puppy pulls on the lid.

⑧ Dab a spot of peanut butter on the door to get your puppy's interest. Tell him "close" and click your clicker the moment he touches the mailbox door. Immediately give him a treat.

⑨ Next, stop clicking him for merely touching the door, and wait for him to push it closed before clicking. Once he is consistently successful, add at third rubber band to your string to hold the door wider open, and finally, remove the rubber bands altogether.

WHAT TO EXPECT: Fetching the mail from the mailbox can be learned in a day or two. Opening and closing the mailbox door can each be learned in about a week.

PUT IT ALL TOGETHER! Familiarize yourself with the process of chaining behaviors (page 154). First teach each of the components, and then chain them together: Your new cue of "get the mail" will come to represent the entire chain.

TROUBLESHOOTING

MY PUPPY OPENS THE MAILBOX DOOR WHEN I WANT HIM TO CLOSE IT

Because all three behaviors use the same prop, you can expect some initial confusion from your puppy as to which behavior he is supposed to do.

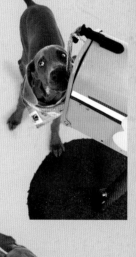

"Treats are probably the best thing in the whole world!"

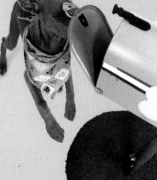

GET THE MAIL

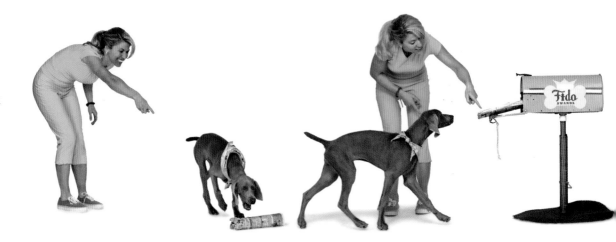

1 Have your puppy fetch the mail from the floor.

2 Place the newspaper exposed in an open mailbox.

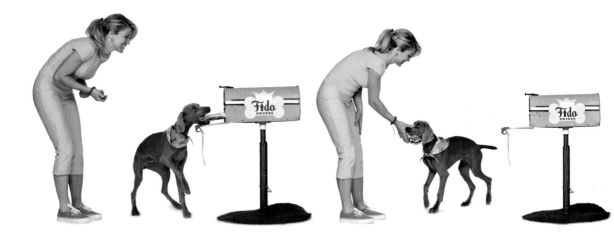

Tell your puppy to "fetch!"

Reward your puppy when he brings it to your hand.

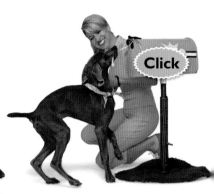

OPEN THE MAILBOX

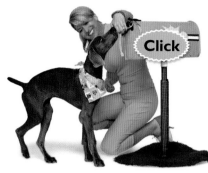
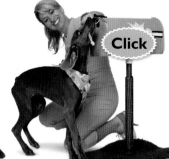

3 Click and reward your puppy for touching the rope.

4 Now wait until your puppy bites the rope before you click.

5 And then challenge your puppy to pull on the rope. Click and reward.

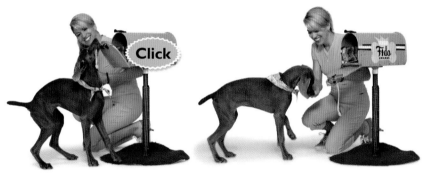

6 Have your puppy pull the mailbox door all the way open. Click and treat.

CLOSE THE MAILBOX

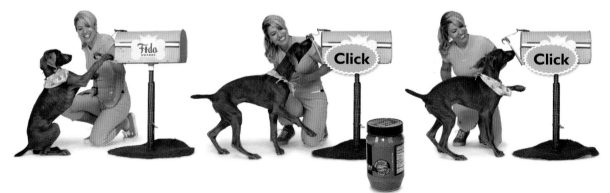

7 Use two rubber bands to hold the mailbox door open.

8 Click when your puppy sniffs the peanut butter on the door.

9 Have your puppy close it completely.

APPENDIX: TRICKS BY SKILL LEVEL

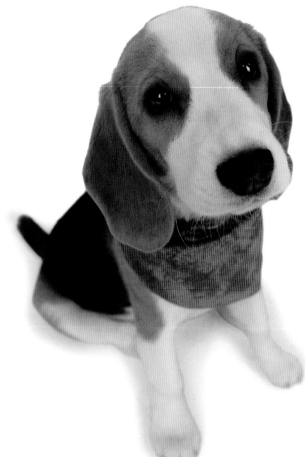

"When I was little
I didn't know any
tricks but now
I already know
three!"

GLOSSARY OF TERMS

Behavior
An action that the puppy performs.

Chaining
The process of combining several behaviors into a continuous sequence.

Clicker
A handheld gadget with a metal tongue that makes a *click-click* sound when pressed. The clicker is commonly used in dog training to make the *reward marker* sound.

Cookie
Dog training vernacular for a treat.

Cue
A word or hand signal that instructs the puppy to perform a behavior.

Luring
The method of using a treat to guide the puppy's head, in an effort to get the puppy to position his body. We can use a treat to lure a puppy in a circle, in order to teach him to "spin."

Marker Training
The method of using a *reward marker* to denote the instant the puppy performs a correct behavior. The exact timing of the reward marker greatly helps the puppy understand what he did to earn the reward. Every reward marker is followed by a treat.

Positive Reinforcement
Positive reinforcement is the rewarding of good behavior in order to increase the behavior; you get your puppy to do a trick, you give him a reward, and he learns to repeat the trick.

Puppy
For the purposes of this book, a puppy is a dog up to two years of age.

Regression
If a puppy has more than two or three unsuccessful attempts in a row, we regress by temporarily lowering the criteria for success. By reverting to an easier step, the puppy can be successful for a while.

Reward
Anything a puppy enjoys (such as praise, play, or a toy) can be used as a reward for good behavior. Treats are the most common reward for puppies.

Reward Marker
A specific unique sound (such as a word or a click from a clicker) that denotes the instant the puppy performs correctly and earns a reward.

Shaping
The method of teaching a trick by breaking it down into baby steps. The most basic component of the trick is rewarded first, then the next component, progressing step-by-step through the entire trick. Reward markers are often used in shaping because they can mark a behavior very precisely.

Training Session
A focused and continuous teaching period. Several five-minute sessions per day are ideal for most puppies.

Treat
A pea-sized soft, tasty food morsel given as a reward or used as a lure.

Treat Bag
Also called a bait bag; a pouch at your waist used to hold treats.

Trick
A behavior performed on cue by the puppy.

Upping the Ante
When we up the ante, we require a more difficult behavior from the puppy than he has previously achieved. As soon as your puppy is achieving a step with about 75 percent success, up the ante and demand a higher skill to earn the treat.

KYRA SUNDANCE

KYRA SUNDANCE'S world-acclaimed acrobatic Stunt Dog Team performs on premier stages internationally at circuses, professional sports halftime shows, and on television shows such as *The Tonight Show*, *Ellen*, *ET*, *Worldwide Fido Awards*, *Animal Planet*, *Showdog Moms & Dads*, and more. Kyra and her dogs starred in Disney's *Underdog* stage show, and starred in a command performance in Marrakech for the King of Morocco. Kyra is nationally ranked in competitive dog sports, has worked as a set trainer for dog actors, and lectures for international professional dog organizations.

Kyra authored several successful books including *101 Dog Tricks* series and the *The Dog Rules*, and starred in several dog tricks DVDs. Kyra and her Weimaraners Chalcy and Jadie live with Kyra's husband on a ranch in California's Mojave Desert. www.kyra.com

JADIE

Jadie (Kyra's Weimaraner puppy) shot the *51 Puppy Tricks* cover photo and many of the full-page trick photos when she was four months old. She shot the step-by step photos when she was between four and five months old. Jadie began her training at the age of eight weeks, performed on Nickelodeon's *Worldwide Fido Awards* at nine weeks, and starred in the *Puppy Tricks* DVD at twenty weeks. We look forward to lots more great things from her as she grows up!

ACKNOWLEDGMENTS

Thanks to Heidi Horn (production assistant, bandanna coordinator, puppy petter, and Kyra's mother), Claire Doré (consultant), and Chalcy (puppy tutor and my own adult Weimaraner). And thanks especially to all the adorable, smart, and talented, puppies: Mabel (bulldog), Luke (Siberian husky), Jamie (dalmatian), Nash (bearded collie), Gibson (white golden retriever), Lucy and Susie (beagles), Dolly and Brody (bloodhounds), and to my own Jadie (Weimaraner puppy).

www.51puppytricks.com

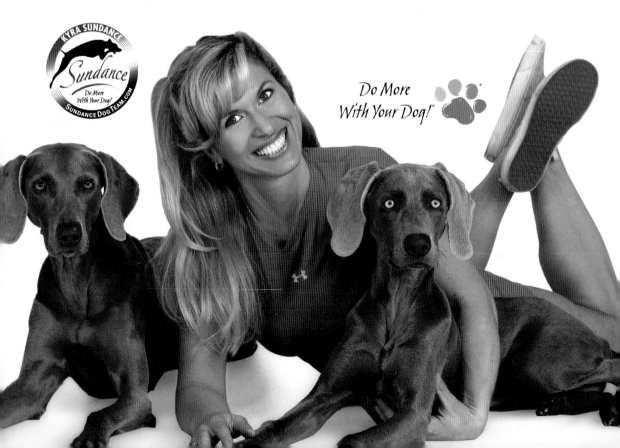

101 DOG TRICKS

STEP-BY-STEP ACTIVITIES TO
ENGAGE, CHALLENGE, AND
BOND WITH YOUR DOG

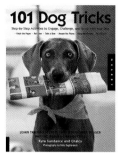

101 Dog Tricks is the
industry standard training
book for adult dogs.
Difficulty ratings range
from "easy" to "expert"
and "build-on" ideas suggest more complicated
tricks that build on each new skill. If you want
to teach your dog to find the remote, carry your
purse, play basketball, and jump rope, this is the
book for you!

THE DOG TRICKS AND TRAINING WORKBOOK

A STEP-BY-STEP INTERACTIVE
CURRICULUM TO ENGAGE,
CHALLENGE, AND BOND
WITH YOUR DOG

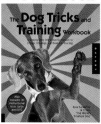

Track your progress as
you work through this
comprehensive curriculum.
Review and *re-evaluation*
sections at the end of each chapter prompt you
to reflect on your progress and your improving
relationship with your dog. Also included: 30
trick cards and a DVD that features step-by-step
instructions for four complete tricks.

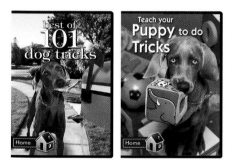

BEST OF 101 DOG TRICKS (DVD)
PUPPY TRICKS (DVD)

STARRING KYRA SUNDANCE

Step-by-step instruction and real world examples
of training a novice dog. The *Puppy Tricks DVD*
contains 17 tricks including: Spin Circles, Open
the Door, Close the Door, Roll Over, Ring a Bell
to Go Outside, Wipe your Paws, Turn on the Tap
Light, and Fetch. The *Dog Tricks DVD* contains 16
tricks including: Say Your Prayers, Jump Through
My Circled Arms, Shake Hands, Crawl, Beg, Take a
Bow, Cover Your Eyes, and Tidy Up Your Toys.

THE DOG RULES

14 SECRETS TO DEVELOPING
THE DOG YOU WANT

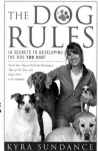

Whether you're frustrated
trying to get through to your
dog; or whether you're looking
to take your training to the
next level; there are concrete
rules that will get you there.
Simple behavior modification techniques such as
"Focus on the Solution, Not the Problem," and
"One Command, One Consequence," empower
owners with a clear strategy. The Dog Rules does
not involve intimidation nor escalating corrections,
but rather fosters a joyful relationship with a dog
who balances enthusiasm with self-control.

ABOUT THE PHOTOGRAPHER: Born in Baltimore, Maryland, Nick Saglimbeni is obsessed with pushing the limits of conventional photography. After earning his Masters degree in Cinematography from the University of Southern California, Nick opened SlickforceStudio, which quickly grew to become one of the most sought-after visual-media studios in Los Angeles. Nick has received three Grand Prize Awards from the National Association of Photoshop Professionals, and he won the 2009 Blackberry Small Business Award. His work has been featured on over 100 magazine covers, and he continues to shoot for TV and film.

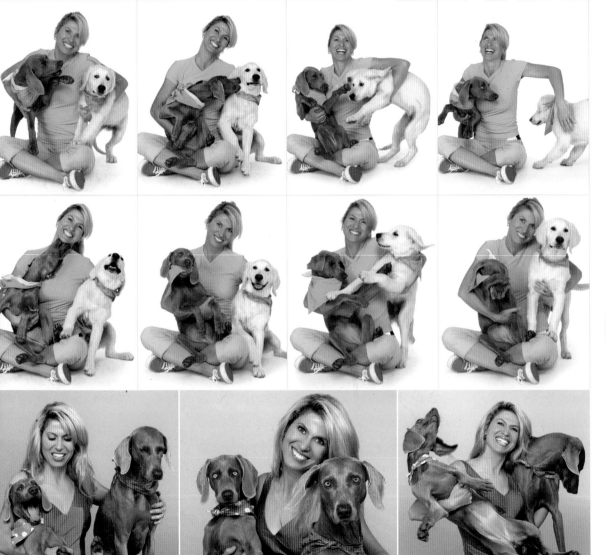